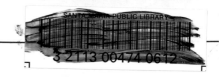
WHAT EXPERTS ARE SAYING ABOUT
The Best Friends Approach to Alzheimer's Care

Best Friends is hard to put down, and will be picked up again and again....This book truly illustrates that good Alzheimer's care can teach us how to care for one another and for ourselves in a way that will make our world a company of best friends.

Jitka Zgola, OT(C), Author, *Doing Things*

I recommend Best Friends highly to anyone who cares for someone with Alzheimer's; it proves life doesn't have to end with a diagnosis.

Burton V. Reifler, M.D., M.P.H.
Professor and Department Chairman, Wake Forest University

The "Best Friends" approach to caring for persons with dementia developed by Troxel and Bell is outstanding! It is practical and full of compassion for persons with dementia and those who care for them.

Joanne Rader, R.N., M.N., F.A.A.N.

Best Friends will become the handbook of choice for families coping with Alzheimer's disease.

Elayne Brill, Founder
Alzheimer's Association—San Francisco Bay Area Chapter

This book is not only a terrific training tool for health care providers, it's an easy-to-understand resource for caregivers who are family and friends.

Rona Smyth Henry, M.B.A., M.P.H.
The Robert Wood Johnson Foundation

A beautifully written book, Best Friends offers a simple but powerful philosophy and model of care that can dramatically change lives. I intend to share this treasure with all who will listen, including families and professionals.

Bonnie Smith, S.S.W., Director,
Board Member, National Adult Day Services Association

...a blueprint for care that can be readily adapted to home, adult day services and residential facilities...If a single book can provide an understanding of how to provide care to people with Alzheimer's disease, this could be it.

Dorothy Seman, R.N., M.S.
Clinical Coordinator, Alzheimer's Family Care Center, Chicago

Bell and Troxel have authored an outstanding manual for AD care....Persons with Alzheimer's and related disorders deserve the type of care outlined in the book—care that is informed, innovative, interpersonal, and individual.

...urnal of Applied Gerontology

The Best Friends
Approach to
Alzheimer's Care

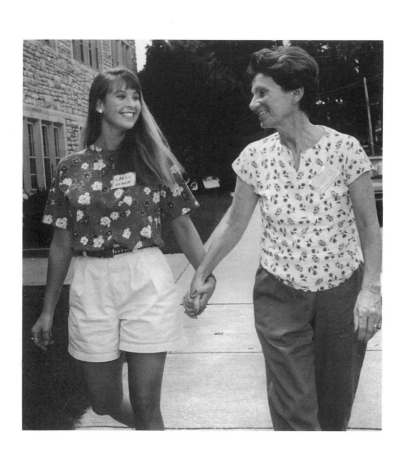

The Best Friends Approach to Alzheimer's Care

Virginia Bell, M.S.W.
and
David Troxel, M.P.H.

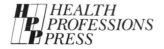
HEALTH PROFESSIONS PRESS

Baltimore • London • Winnipeg • Sydney

Health Professions Press, Inc.
Post Office Box 10624
Baltimore, Maryland 21285-0624

www.healthpropress.com

Cover design by James V. McCabe, Four Winds Productions, Baltimore, Maryland.
Manufactured in the United States of America by Thomson-Shore, Dexter, Michigan.

First printing, November 1996   Third printing, April 1999
Second printing, September 1997   Fourth printing, November 2000

Photo credit: p. ii—Carrie Kenady (left) and Geri Greenway (right) take a walk outside the Alzheimer's Association Helping Hand Day Center, Lexington, Kentucky (courtesy of and copyright © 1993, Mark Cornelison and *The Lexington Herald-Leader*).

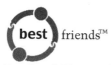 friends™

Best Friends™ is a trademark owned by Health Professions Press, Inc.

Library of Congress Cataloging-in-Publication Data
Bell, Virginia.
The best friends approach to Alzheimer's care / Virginia Bell, David Troxel.
    p. cm.
  Includes bibliographical references and index.
  ISBN 1-878812-35-1
  1. Alzheimer's disease—Patients—Long-term care.   I. Troxel, David.   II. Title.
RC523.B43 1996
362.1′96831—dc20
                                                              96-23307
                                                              CIP

British Library Cataloguing in Publication Data are available from the British Library.

Contents

Acknowledgments

Because this book represents so much of our experience and work since the mid-1980s, there are many people to thank who have guided us with their advice and wisdom and in some cases reviewed sections of this book.

Many at the Sanders-Brown Center on Aging of the University of Kentucky deserve special acknowledgment. Dr. William Markesbery, Center Director, motivated us with his insistence that the best treatment for Alzheimer's disease is loving care. Dr. David Wekstein first brought us together as colleagues and guided us through many of our early experiences in support groups and Alzheimer's care. Other Sanders-Brown faculty and staff provided us with ideas, inspiration, and friendship, including Dr. Linda Kuder, Dr. Deborah Danner, and Marie Smart.

The Board of Directors and staff of the Lexington/Bluegrass Chapter of the Alzheimer's Association were early pioneers in direct services and in the development of the Helping Hand Day Center and In-Home Program. We would like to offer particular thanks to Sherry Kyker, Sharon Reed, and past board members Claire Macfarlane, Marie Masters, Jane Owen, Margaret Patterson, and Ray Rector and association staff members Joan Skillman, Robin Hamon Kern, Patricia McCray, Barry McDaniels, Gwyn Rubio, and Tonya Tincher.

The Board of Directors of the Santa Barbara Chapter of the Alzheimer's Association believed in this project and supported its Executive Director in his taking time to write this book. Special thanks go to Barbara Browne and Charles Zimmer; board members Elayne Brill, Louise Davis, Inge Gatz, Selma Rubin, Carmen K. Singh, and Jeanne West; and association staff members Stephanie Smagala, Marge Collins, Debbie McConnell, Ellen Moggia, Anna Marie Weiner, and Dianne Timmerman.

Many staff, volunteers, and families at AD Care Adult Day Centers, part of LifeSpan Services Network, Inc., of San Luis Obispo County, California, were influential in this project, especially Pam Richards, Susan Bailey, and Bev Faldalen. Alyce Crawford, of the Coast Caregiver Resource

Center of San Luis Obispo County, is a "local hero" for her always-creative solutions for the most difficult problems.

Many staff members of the national Alzheimer's Association have been wonderful sounding boards over the years. Particular thanks go to Tom Kirk and Sam Fazio of the Association's Patient and Family Services staff.

We also acknowledge the outstanding contributions of individuals who have been mentors to us in the field of Alzheimer's disease research and practice, including Lisa Gwyther of Duke University, Dr. Miriam Aronson of the Institute on Aging at the Bergin Pines County Hospital, and Dr. Robert Katzman of the University of California, San Diego.

We thank Dr. Steven DeKosky of the University of Pittsburgh Alzheimer's Disease Research Center for his continued support over the years.

The Robert Wood Johnson Foundation, through its Dementia Care & Respite Services Program, co-funded by the national Alzheimer's Association and the federal Administration on Aging, has helped launch the adult day center movement. We thank this foundation for its support of our work in the Helping Hand program, with a particular acknowledgment to Rona Smyth Henry at the Foundation, and Dr. Burton V. Reifler and Nancy J. Cox at the National Program Office at Bowman Gray School of Medicine of Wake Forest University.

Other foundations and organizations have made contributions to our work by giving funds to put many of these ideas into practice. Special thanks go to the Steele-Reese Foundation, the Wood-Claeyssens Foundation, and the National Association of Retired Federal Employees.

Dr. Linda Hewett of the University of California, San Francisco, Alzheimer's Disease Center of Central California, reviewed this manuscript and provided comments on sexuality that are included in Chapter 7. Drs. Robert Harbaugh and Erno Daniel of Santa Barbara reviewed Chapter 3.

Finally, a few personal acknowledgments:

From Virginia Bell—To the many Helping Hand volunteers who have exemplified the Best Friends model since 1984; and to my husband, Wayne Bell, and our children and grandchildren who have had to live with a nontraditional wife, mother, and grandmother in order for this book to be published.

From David Troxel—To my parents Fred and Dorothy Troxel, who have provided wonderful love and support; to Dr. Audrey Gotsch, a friend and mentor, who taught me that even vexing problems have solutions; and to Betty Branch, Robert Fluno, Mary Jo Jones, and Ronald Spingarn.

*To the many persons with Alzheimer's disease
who have inspired us with their courage,
and to their caregivers, who have inspired us
with their commitment, wisdom, and loving care.*

Introduction

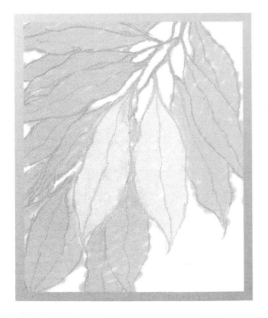

The Best Friends Approach to Alzheimer's Care reflects a growing optimism in the field of Alzheimer's care that much can be done to improve the lives of people with the disease and to transform caregiving from a terrible burden to care that is manageable. The book represents the development of the first comprehensive model of care, which is easy to understand and learn. With the Best Friends model of care, readers will be able to develop the know-how, what we call the "knack," of responding to any situation. This book demonstrates that the secret of good Alzheimer's care is not necessarily in what is done, it is in the doing.

The authors have over 20 years of combined national and international experience at university research centers, Alzheimer's Association chapters, adult day services centers, support groups, classrooms, and home settings. We have lectured in 15 states and nine countries. We have spent thousands of hours, one-on-one, with persons who have Alzheimer's disease and their caregivers. We have been through the frontier days of Alzheimer's care.

In the early 1980s almost no educational materials were available, and there were even fewer services for individuals with dementia and their families. As that decade progressed, a network of family support groups developed into a strong and vital national Alzheimer's Association. In 1987 the respected Robert Wood Johnson Foundation committed millions of dollars to a national initiative to study adult day services for people with dementia and to encourage their development.

In the 1990s there has been continued expansion of adult day services programs, continued growth of the Alzheimer's Association and its chapter network, and a growing trend to provide more services to and therapeutic interventions for the *individual* with dementia. More and more people are being diagnosed with Alzheimer's disease very early; this trend will change the face of Alzheimer's care. A milestone came in late 1994 when former U.S. President Ronald Reagan courageously announced his diagnosis of Alzheimer's disease.

In looking back, we can celebrate our successes. Enormous strides in research, diagnostic standards, family services, and public awareness have been made. Yet, despite these successes, many families and professionals we talk to are in trouble. They tell us that problem behaviors still create enormous difficulties, that nursing assistants are inadequately trained, that planned activities fall flat, and that it is still a struggle to make it through the day.

The Best Friends model addresses these problems by going beyond a laundry list of tips. Readers will learn a model of caregiving, a way of approaching the challenges, that will work for the betterment of both family and professional caregivers.

This book differs from other books in the field in a number of ways. First, the authors have adopted a positive, optimistic outlook. We believe that too much attention has been paid to the "tragic" side of Alzheimer's disease; our collection of books and pamphlets on Alzheimer's disease includes negative labels such as "victim," "the funeral that never ends," "the mean stage," "the living death," and "the worse fate." We understand the enormous weight that Alzheimer's disease places on caregiving individuals and families. This is a terrible disease. Yet, by dwelling on the negative, it is too easy to victimize people with the illness and settle for lower standards of care. Caregivers, too, can be victimized by this attitude, this assumption that they are all helpless and hopeless.

Second, all family stories mentioned in this book are real, and include the full names of the people involved. We do this to reduce the stigma of Alzheimer's disease, to bring it out of the darkness. We worried that families would be uncomfortable with this technique, but when we asked them for written permission to tell their stories, they all said yes. They did this to remember or honor their loved ones and to support a greater understanding of Alzheimer's disease. We commend them for their openness and encourage the reader to learn more about the family members in Appendix C.

Third, the focus of this book is on individuals with Alzheimer's disease, what they are experiencing, and how to help them. By putting the spotlight on the individual with dementia, we are not in any way negating the impact of Alzheimer's disease on the caregiver. We know that it affects the whole family and that caregivers are often at great risk for premature disability and death. However, if we can improve the quality of life and behavior of people with Alzheimer's disease, by definition we have also improved the life of the caregiver. Alzheimer's disease care need not be debilitating.

This book covers the full spectrum of Alzheimer's care using the Best Friends model.

Chapter 1 describes the experience of Alzheimer's disease. We believe it is important to understand what it is like to have Alzheimer's disease to become a better, more empathetic, caregiver.

Chapter 2 offers a short primer on Alzheimer's disease called "The Basics."

Chapter 3 tells the reader how to make an assessment of the individual's strengths and abilities. This assessment is important for setting appropriate expectations and planning good care.

Chapter 4 introduces the Alzheimer's Disease Bill of Rights. It is the underlying philosophy behind the book and argues that we must all strive for the best quality of care and quality of life for the person with dementia.

Chapter 5 reveals how the art of good friendship teaches us much about good Alzheimer's care. It suggests that recasting relationships can make caregiving easier and more rewarding for families and professionals. In this chapter we introduce many of "our friends," persons with Alzheimer's disease or related disorders whose stories we tell.

Chapter 6 reviews the importance of the affected individual's life story, cultural background, and traditions to good-quality care.

Chapter 7 brings together all of the ingredients of the Best Friends model of care and introduces our concept of the "knack" of caregiving.

Chapter 8 describes the knack of communicating. We offer a number of "dos" and "don'ts" that will be helpful to the caregiver.

Chapter 9 examines the knack of activities, noting the importance of getting away from "programming activities" and, instead, making them a natural part of each day. This chapter is of particular interest to adult day centers and long-term care facilities, but can also help home caregivers.

Chapters 10, 11, and 12 present examples of the Best Friends model in action, showing how it can be applied to home care, adult day center care, and care in long-term facilities. Of particular interest to adult day centers and long-term care facilities is the discussion in Chapter 11 about involving volunteers in Alzheimer's care.

Chapter 13 challenges caregivers to be their own best friends. Taking even simple steps can reduce stress and strain. Even better, the Best Friends model can bring joy back into the caregiver's life.

Chapter 14 offers a few final thoughts on being a Best Friend to a *person* with Alzheimer's disease, and shows how negative feelings, which are normal, can be turned into positive feelings. Light *can* come out of darkness.

Appendix A contains a listing of national and local resources for individuals with dementia and their caregivers. Appendix B provides a list of suggested readings. Appendix C offers brief biographies of the individuals with Alzheimer's disease or related disorders whose stories we tell in this book.

We believe this book will help readers in a number of ways: *Families* reading this book will gain a renewed sense of hope. The Best Friends model encourages families to rethink their approach to care; techniques and suggestions are offered to invigorate their efforts to offer effective, loving care.

Nursing facility staff reading this book will find easy, simple-to-use methods in the care of residents with dementia. The Best Friends model lends itself to staff training and can be easily learned and understood by today's multicultural staff, who may also have differing educational backgrounds. Included are ideas for activities that can be used during almost any interaction with a resident. Because the Best Friends model emphasizes the importance of an upbeat, positive approach, the model also will improve staff morale and family satisfaction.

Adult day center staff who adopt the Best Friends model will learn methods that can enrich center programming and attract greater numbers of volunteers. The book also discusses how the Best Friends model can help centers with one of their most vexing problems—convincing families to utilize this needed service.

Finally, *individuals* diagnosed with emerging Alzheimer's disease may gain insight from reading this book. We hope that these readers will share our vision that their quality of life can still be good even when facing the enormous challenge presented by Alzheimer's disease.

In conclusion, we would like to draw readers' attention to the following points:

1. Although this book addresses Alzheimer's disease, the concepts apply to any individual with irreversible dementing disorder. Thus individuals and families coping with multi-infarct dementia (mini-strokes) or dementia caused by Parkinson's disease, AIDS, or other disorders can benefit from the Best Friends model.

2. This book does not examine research and medical treatment issues in depth, in part because information in these areas changes rapidly in the contemporary research environment. Local Alzheimer's Association newsletters and national Alzheimer's Association publications are the best sources for current information on research and treatment. We do offer information on the basics of Alzheimer's disease in Chapter 2 to provide the reader with an understanding of fundamental principles of these issues.

3. The authors believe that the literature on Alzheimer's disease has long been overdependent on the use of "stages" to describe the disease. Alzheimer's disease is a *process*, a continuum of illness. It is not helpful to pigeonhole someone into any one stage because every case is different. As we once heard a neurologist say, "If you've met one person with Alzheimer's disease, you've only met one person with Alzheimer's disease."

4. We coin a new phrase in this book, *emerging Alzheimer's disease,* to describe the growing number of people with Alzheimer's disease who are diagnosed early enough to be able to have a significant say in their care and future. We describe the progression of

the disease in a simple fashion as emerging, early, middle, and late Alzheimer's disease.

5.   We describe nursing facilities or board and care homes as *long-term care facilities* or simply as *facilities*. We describe adult day care centers as *adult day services*, *adult day centers*, or simply *centers*.

6.   All authors writing about dementia struggle with the question of how to describe the man or woman with dementia. We reject labels such as "Alzheimer's victim," "memory-affected individual," and "Alzheimer's person" because they collapse the person into the pathology of the disease. The word "patient" only applies to the settings in which an individual is being seen by a medical professional. Neutral phrases such as "the person with Alzheimer's disease," "those with dementia," and "the person with memory loss," become bulky and laborious for the reader. In this book, we will use *person(s)* to describe individual(s) with Alzheimer's disease or a related disorder. We hope this will be more economical to the reader than other phrasing. At the same time, this term gently reminds us that there is a *person* beneath the cloak of dementia, one who has feelings, one who has led a life full of rich experiences, and one who deserves dignified care.

I

About
Alzheimer's
Disease

The experience of Alzheimer's

disease, basic information every

family and professional caregiver

should know, and the ways in

which to make a basic assessment

of the person's strengths and

abilities in order to set appropriate

expectations

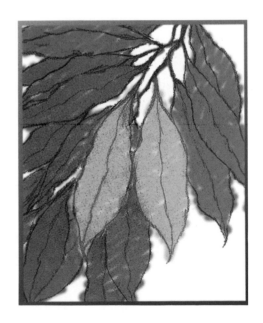

1

The Experience of Alzheimer's Disease

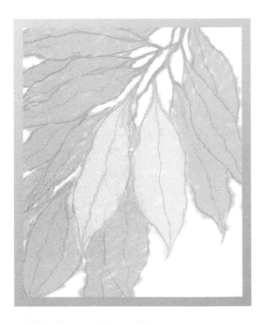

When the authors began helping people with Alzheimer's disease and their caregivers, we asked: What is it like to have Alzheimer's disease? What is it like to be unsure of one's surroundings, to have difficulty communicating, not to recognize a once-familiar face, or to be unable to do things one has always enjoyed?

We imagined that the experience of Alzheimer's disease might be similar to taking a long trip in a foreign country. The language is puzzling. Customs are different. How does the pay phone work? Ordering food in a restaurant proves difficult. When paying a restaurant bill with unfamiliar currency, the traveler might fear being shortchanged, cheated. Tasks so easy at home are major challenges in an unfamiliar setting.

The *person* with Alzheimer's disease is in a foreign land all the time. He or she experiences culture shock even in his or her own backyard (Figure 1).

A growing number of individuals are diagnosed early in the disease process with *emerging* Alzheimer's disease. These individuals represent a new type of "client" for service providers. Support groups are no longer just for caregivers but also for people with the disease. Conferences no longer feature only caregivers telling their stories; some feature talks given by people diagnosed with Alzheimer's disease. One *person* with emerging Alzheimer's disease told the authors her story.

Rebecca Riley, a nurse and educator, was diagnosed with Alzheimer's disease in 1984 at age 59. When she began having difficulty teaching, she thought it was because the course content was new. Soon she knew something was wrong with her thinking and memory, and she suspected that she might have Alzheimer's disease. A medical examination later confirmed her suspicions.

Rebecca was our first teacher about the world of Alzheimer's disease. Some written notes she made describing her experience included the following:

- *Depression.*
- *Can't say what I want.*
- *Afraid I can't express my thoughts and words—thus I remain silent and become depressed.*
- *I need conversation to be slowly.*
- *It is difficult to follow conversation with so much noise.*
- *I feel that people turn me off because I cannot express myself.*
- *I dislike social workers, nurses & friends who do not treat me as a real person.*
- *It is difficult to live one day at a time. My philosophy adopted July 30, 1984.*

Reading Rebecca's heartfelt words, one can begin to understand the experience of Alzheimer's disease. She knows that she is losing her language skills and ability to communicate her wishes. Her writing reveals that her once-meticulous grammar is slipping. Complexity is her enemy; she cannot follow the din and roar of competing conversations—she calls it "the noise."

Her statement about social workers, nurses, and friends who do not treat her as a "real person" may make the reader both smile and wince. Even though her cognitive skills are in decline, she senses correctly that people are treating her differently. Consequently, she feels anger and some resentment toward these people.

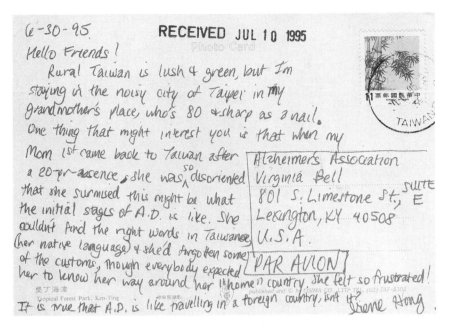

6-30-95

RECEIVED JUL 10 1995

Photo Card

Hello Friends!

Rural Taiwan is lush & green, but I'm staying in the noisy city of Taipei in my grandmother's place, who's 80 & sharp as a nail. One thing that might interest you is that when my Mom 1st came back to Taiwan after a 20-yr absence, she was so disoriented that she surmised this might be what the initial stages of A.D. is like. She couldn't find the right words in Taiwanese (her native language) & she'd forgotten some of the customs, though everybody expected her to know her way around her "home" country. She felt so frustrated! It is true that A.D. is like travelling in a foreign country, isn't it?

Alzheimer's Association
Virginia Bell
801 S. Limestone St., Suite E
Lexington, KY 40508
U.S.A.

[PAR AVION]

Irene Hong

Figure 1. Postcard from student Irene Hong, who volunteered in the Helping Hand of Lexington, Kentucky, for a year. She is studying to be a neurologist.

Remarkably, she is trying to create a plan for the future. She decides to take things "one day at a time." As evident in her notes, she struggles to do this, acknowledging that this will be difficult. Yet, she adopts it as her "personal philosophy," and even puts in the date to somehow formalize and legalize the decision. It is as if her nursing background reminded her of the importance of documenting such decisions in writing, for the record.

Rebecca's shared insight into her own illness is helpful as we try to understand the experience of having Alzheimer's disease. Without understanding her world, we cannot possibly develop a successful strategy for improving her quality of care and her quality of life.

COMMON EMOTIONS AND FEELINGS OF PERSONS WITH ALZHEIMER'S DISEASE

Every *person's* response to Alzheimer's Disease is different, but many people will experience one or more of the emotions listed in Table 1.

Table 1.   Common emotions and feelings of *persons* with Alzheimer's disease

Loss	Frustration
Isolation and loneliness	Fear
Sadness	Paranoia
Confusion	Anger
Worry and anxiety	Embarrassment

Loss

Many people define themselves in large part by their jobs, their relationships, or the things they do. One might say, "I am proud to be a good carpenter," "I am Wayne's mother/father," or "I am a fly fisherman." If any of us had to make a major change in life and these roles were taken from us, we would experience feelings of great loss. People with Alzheimer's disease lose these titles and, as a result, lose these important and meaningful roles. Eventually, they will be unable to work, and will have to give up favorite activities such as driving a car or preparing a meal, symbols of independence. Sooner or later, the losses mount.

Rebecca Riley was aware of her losses. She said, "Of course you know you're the first to know."

Isolation and Loneliness

A friend of the authors broke his leg in a skiing accident and had to curtail most of his activities for a month. He could not go to the office, could not work out at the gym, gave up his opera tickets, and had to cancel outings with friends. He told us that he was very lonely during his recuperation. His first day back at work was one of the happiest of his life. "Thank goodness I no longer have to watch daytime television!" he exclaimed to his co-workers.

As Alzheimer's disease progresses, *persons* often feel increasingly isolated. They can no longer drive and may no longer be able to play their weekly bridge game, go sailing with friends, do woodworking, go shopping, or even walk down to the neighborhood donut shop. They lose social contacts; worse yet, friends eventually stop visiting them. Unlike a broken leg, their memory cannot be mended.

Other factors can lead to isolation and loneliness. The many daily tasks faced by caregivers, such as personal care, housekeeping, bill paying, and other chores, may shorten time that can be spent with the *person*. Moving away from a hometown to be closer to family members can further isolate the *person* from longtime friends.

A former teacher and community leader, Rubena Dean often felt left out of activities. She once said, "I used to play cards, I used to drive, I used to work . . . there are too many 'used tos' in my life now."

Sadness

Everyone becomes sad about some event—small or large—in life. Feelings of sadness can walk hand-in-hand with Alzheimer's disease, particularly for individuals with emerging Alzheimer's disease, who are often aware of what lies ahead. (*Note:* A brief discussion of depression and Alzheimer's disease is found on page 22.)

Geri Greenway was at the peak of her career as a college professor when she was diagnosed with Alzheimer's disease in her late 40s. Aware of the nature of the disease, she often sat with her hands covering her eyes, as if her world was too painful to see.

Rebecca Riley's list begins with the single word "Depression." Then she writes, "Afraid I can't express my thoughts and words—thus I remain silent and become depressed."

Confusion

All of us become confused now and then. Perhaps an always-dependable friend does not show up for a lunch date. Could it be that we have gone to different restaurants? Maybe one of us got the time and date mixed up. For many people with Alzheimer's disease, confusion is a daily, even hourly, experience. The *person* is never quite sure about anything—the time of day, the place, and the people around him or her.

Larkin Myers was at home watching the Winter Olympics on television when he became confused. Just as he observed a high-speed toboggan cross the finish line, his wife, Chris, walked in front of the television. He gasped and exclaimed, "You, you drove that contraption?" When his wife looked puzzled, he insisted, "You just arrived in that thing, didn't you?" Next week, the support group gave Chris a "gold medal" in the Olympics of Caregiving.

Worry and Anxiety

We all worry sometimes. Parents may worry about their teenage child who is not home by curfew. Families may worry about having enough money to pay all the bills at the end of the month. Some people may even worry that a favorite celebrity's marriage is in trouble after reading the latest tabloid at the supermarket! We can also experience moments of free-floating anxiety. Maybe we cannot quite name it, but we may often or occasionally feel anxious.

The *person* with Alzheimer's disease can become consumed by worry and anxiety. One frequent by-product of dementia is that the *person* cannot separate a small worry from an all-consuming concern. For example, a *person* at a nursing facility begins worrying about dark clouds in the sky seen through a window. Left unchecked, the worry can wreck his or her afternoon and as a result, the afternoon of the people around him or her.

Willa McCabe, a retired elementary schoolteacher, often worried about the children in her classes. "I'm late for school. I have to go now. The children are waiting for me," she would insist, although she had stopped working more than a dozen years earlier.

People with emerging Alzheimer's disease may worry about what lies ahead.

Rebecca Riley worried about what lay ahead. Referring to a book on Alzheimer's disease, she said, "I know what happens. I've read the end of The 36-Hour Day.[1] *I'm a nurse, you know."*

Frustration

We all have known the frustration of misplacing our car keys, which makes us late for work or for an appointment. We know they are in the house but we cannot find them. Imagine the frustration of losing one's keys or wallet every day, every hour. The *person* with Alzheimer's disease may constantly be looking for something he or she is certain is lost.

Frustration may also stem from failing to complete everyday tasks. In the morning a thoughtful caregiver may leave clothes on the bed for the woman with Alzheimer's disease to whom she provides

---

[1] A revised edition was published in 1991; see Appendix B.

care. The woman stares at the pile—hose, underwear, a slip, a blouse, a skirt, a sweater, shoes, and jewelry—what goes on first?, she wonders. What may have been so simple once is actually an elaborate series of steps performed in a certain sequence: put on the hose before the shoes, the bra before the blouse. Yet, because she often loses her ability to sequence, this woman with Alzheimer's disease may find that even the act of dressing can lead to great frustration.

Accustomed to using his reasoning and problem-solving abilities in his work, Brevard Crihfield, the former executive director of the Council of State Governments, summed up his experience of Alzheimer's disease when he said in frustration, "It is like my head is a big knob turned to off."

Fear

The authors spoke to a friend who had driven her car into New York City to attend a Broadway play. She had found a parking space on the street to save money, but after the show realized that she had forgotten the exact location of her car. She described her search for the car and her growing sense of fear and panic. The street was deserted. Did she hear footsteps behind her? What if the car had been stolen? Forgetting a car's location could happen to anyone. She was genuinely afraid for her personal safety. Part of her fear was imagined; there were no footsteps behind her.

Persons with Alzheimer's disease may live in fear that is real or imagined. Common fearful thoughts include "Someone has taken my money" or, at the day center, "Will my son pick me up today?" They may feel fear about the future, the loss of independence, or the guilt that they are placing too much burden on family members. Sometimes fear can be caused by the fact that dementia can affect visuospatial perceptions. These perceptions may cause, for example, a genuine fear of falling because the carpeting on the floor has a confusing or misleading pattern.

Fear can be one reason the *person* does not want to bathe. A *person* may not want to disrobe in front of someone whom he or she does not remember having met before. Simple things associated with bathing, such as the sound of running water and being immersed in the water, are all potentially quite frightening.

Alzheimer's disease often made Ruby Lee Chiles fearful. During even a simple (and safe) game at the adult day center, she often commented, "Someone is going to get hurt."

The world of a *person* with dementia can be scary.

Paranoia

Many of us have known moments of paranoia. If a boss has been treating an employee differently in the last few weeks, that employee may wonder if the boss is unhappy with his or her performance and is about to fire him or her. A person may be suspicious if there is no mail 2 days in a row. Is someone taking the mail? Is it being lost at the post office?

People with Alzheimer's disease often look for an explanation about what is happening to them. Why does their family refuse to let them drive? Where is their money? If they cannot find rational explanations, they might imagine that someone is trying to harm or hurt them in some way. They may have a delusion, or fixed, false idea, that their child or spouse is a stranger trying to hurt them.

Ruby Mae Morris always made it a point to dress appropriately and fashionably. She enjoyed dressing up for a special occasion. As her dementia worsened, she thought often about her wardrobe. She sometimes became paranoid about the possibility that someone had taken her nice clothes.

Anger

All of us get angry occasionally. Some people "fly off the handle" at the slightest provocation. Others may become angry only when pushed to the limit of their patience. Some people may never get angry even when they should. Sadly, some people let their anger translate into violence. Yet anger has a constructive purpose in life. It can help one fight a battle if threatened. It can release harmful stress and emotion. Also, sometimes "getting something off your chest," becoming angry, can lead to healing in relationships.

It is a myth that all, or even most, people with Alzheimer's disease are violent. Yet people with dementia can become angry because they may not always understand what is happening around them and to them. These reactions may begin with frustration and, if left unchecked, turn to anger.

Anger can be self-directed. For example, a *person* who had been an accountant might sit down to balance his or her checkbook or work on income taxes only to struggle to get the sums to balance. The *person* knows something is wrong, and may become frustrated and angry at his or her inability to do something that was once so easy. Sometimes the anger is directed at others, even the most caring family member.

Thelma Moody's family coined a phrase, "intimate companionship," for their caregiving efforts. Thelma responds well to physical touch, to music, to stories read to her, and simply to be with her family. And, being human, Thelma sometimes becomes frightened or angry.

Embarrassment

All of us can remember a time in school when the teacher called on us and we did not know the answer to a question. How did we feel? We remember the feeling of our collar tightening, voice faltering, palms sweating, and face blushing.

The *person* with Alzheimer's disease is in a giant classroom every day, one in which he or she never has the exact answer.

Because of his shy nature, Vern Clark would sometimes become embarrassed when he could not express himself well at the day center. Fortunately, the staff and volunteers knew how to give him the support he needed. When he experienced a difficult moment, a staff member might say, "What I admire most about you, Vern, is your creativity!" or "Don't worry. I get those things mixed up, too!" Hearing these statements allowed Vern to recover quickly from any embarrassment.

The Best Friends model helps us understand that all the feelings expressed by people with dementia are normal. The power of the model is that good friendship and loving care can minimize negative feelings and have a positive impact on behavior and daily life.

CONCLUSION

After reading this chapter, readers are encouraged to imagine what it is like to have Alzheimer's disease. Table 1 lists some of the common emotions. Using the simple worksheet "The Experience of Alzheimer's Disease" (p. 18) readers can make their own lists of what they think the *person* with Alzheimer's disease is experiencing.

THE EXPERIENCE
OF ALZHEIMER'S DISEASE

How would I feel if I were diagnosed with Alzheimer's disease?

_____

_____

_____

_____

_____

_____

_____

_____

What is the *person* I care about experiencing?

_____

_____

_____

_____

_____

_____

_____

_____

Another simple exercise can help readers begin to understand the impact of this disease: Take 10 small pieces of paper. On each piece, write one of your favorite activities. A typical activity might be visiting the grandchildren, taking a day trip in the car, enjoying a favorite hobby, going to work, trying a new recipe, playing golf, or talking on the phone with an old friend. After you are through, select an activity, think about how much you enjoy it, and then imagine giving it up. Take the piece of paper listing the activity, wad it up, and throw it away. Continue to do this until you have discarded all 10 pieces. How do you feel?

If any of us experienced memory or judgment problems, if any of us was afraid of something, if any of us had to give up most or all of his or her favorite activities, it would be perfectly *normal* to be depressed or anxious, to hide things, to wander away from a possibly threatening situation, or to strike out at someone we think is trying to hurt us.

As the saying goes, to understand someone, we must sometimes "walk a mile in his shoes." When we walk this mile—or run this marathon, as many caregivers may feel—we begin to see one of the underlying surprises of this book: The so-called inappropriate behaviors of Alzheimer's disease are not all that mysterious.

We must think about the experience of Alzheimer's disease and the impact it has on the *person*. This is the starting point for learning to provide the best quality of care for the *person* with Alzheimer's disease. Also, because the *person's* medical condition will not change, as caregivers, *we* must change.

Whether one is caring for someone at home; is a long-distance caregiver; or works in a nursing facility, adult day center, or other professional setting, the Best Friends model of care will show how to respond to most situations and will provide techniques that will prevent or reduce many of the behaviors that cause the most trouble. The result is not only an improvement in the *person's* quality of life, but an improvement in one's own well-being.

2

Alzheimer's Disease Basics

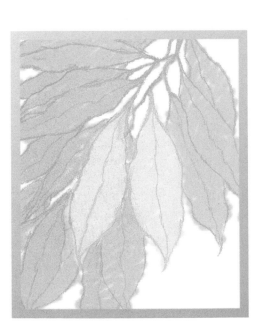

The Best Friends model of care does not depend upon caregivers becoming experts on the medical or scientific aspects of the disease. However, some basic concepts about Alzheimer's disease and caregiving are important to understand in order to implement the Best Friends model. For additional information on medical management, diagnosis, and research, or any of the topics discussed in this chapter, the reader is referred to the select readings in Appendix B. Also, each chapter of the national Alzheimer's Association has a wealth of specialized brochures, books, videos, and other materials that are free or available for a modest charge.

A few basic, but important, concepts about Alzheimer's disease must be understood in order to provide the best quality of care.

OVERVIEW

Significant memory loss, a decline in problem-solving ability, changes in personality and mood, problems with language, and a decline in initiative or "get up and go" are all signs that someone may have Alzheimer's disease, or some other form of dementia. Many things can cause *dementia,* which is often defined as a decline in intellectual functioning that is severe enough to interfere with an individual's ability to carry out usual, day-to-day tasks. Symptoms of dementia, such as significant memory loss, decline in judgment, unusual personality changes, or loss of initiative, are not a part of normal aging.

Persons with Alzheimer's disease are not mentally ill, are not faking symptoms, and are not just being stubborn.

The progression of Alzheimer's disease affects selected areas of the brain, which explains in part why the *person* retains some skills and loses others. For example, the ability to speak is located in a different part of the brain than the ability to sing; thus many people with dementia retain their ability to remember lyrics and sing songs even after their spoken language skills diminish. Also, behaviors that we think are strange, unusual, or upsetting are often the *person's* way of coping with a world that is real to him or her. For example, when a *person* hides his or her car keys and wallet, it is actually a normal action any of us might take if we believed someone was trying to steal our valuables.

DIAGNOSIS

When the symptoms of dementia occur, it is important to gain a full understanding of the underlying cause, whether it be Alzheimer's disease or another cause such as stroke, Parkinson's disease, Huntington's disease, or Pick's disease. It is important to know the underlying cause in order for the *person* to receive the best and most appropriate care. A medical evaluation can reveal a problem that mimics Alzheimer's disease and that may be treatable, even reversible, if detected early. Many causes of dementia are treatable, including depression, thyroid problems, drug interactions, and nutritional deficits.

Depression can mimic many symptoms of Alzheimer's disease and can be a common excess disability in *persons* with dementia. It is treatable with counseling and/or medications. A thorough medical evaluation always takes into consideration the possibility of depression.

Alzheimer's disease cannot be diagnosed by simple observation. A *complete workup* should be done by a competent physician and should include 1) a good medical history; 2) a general physical examination; 3) a neurological examination, which gauges nervous system problems by measuring the individual's gait, eye movement, and reflexes; and 4) a number of laboratory tests (e.g., blood count, blood chemistry), which may indicate potential abnormalities such as infections, anemia, too-high or too-low thyroid levels, or too low vitamin B12 levels. Testing may also include a computerized tomography (CT) or other scan to look for problems such as stroke, hydrocephalus, or tumors. Less frequently, an electroencephalogram (EEG) is done to look for abnormal brain wave activity, which can reveal problems such as epilepsy.

A *neuropsychological test* should be done, which may include written tests and interviews to assess the extent of cognitive decline. Detailed neuropsychological testing can reveal deficits even when the patient is skilled at covering up his or her symptoms. A *psychiatric evaluation* is also sometimes advised to look for depression or other mental illness that may be responsible for, or contribute to, the *person's* dementia.

Although in 1996 there is no definitive test for Alzheimer's disease, families should have confidence in the diagnosis made by a practitioner familiar with evaluating dementia. Treatable causes of dementia are almost never missed if the evaluation is carefully performed.

KEY SERVICES TO CONSIDER AFTER A DIAGNOSIS OF ALZHEIMER'S DISEASE

Families should seek *competent legal counsel,* possibly from an attorney specializing in elder law, to make appropriate legal and financial plans. Priority should be assigned to obtaining durable power of attorney documents that cover finances and health care. These documents allow an appointed representative (typically a family member) to make financial and health care decisions for the *person.* The power of attorney for finances can be abused if given to an unreliable party, so families should proceed with caution.

Families also should learn about *local agencies* that can provide help, notably the nearest chapter of the Alzheimer's Association. The services of an *adult day center* should be utilized if possible, because this type of program can be helpful to the individual with dementia and can give the caregiver a break from care (*respite care*). In addition, families should attend an area *Alzheimer's disease support group* to learn more about the disease and make connections with other caregivers.

RESEARCH NEWS

Increasing numbers of drugs that may improve cognitive functioning and better manage extreme behaviors are already becoming more accessible. The family should stay informed about research by attending conferences and workshops and reading Alzheimer's Association newsletters. Many university research centers and some private physicians are engaged in experimental drug research. This research should be vigorously investigated by individuals and families, particularly when the *person* has emerging or early Alzheimer's disease.

Announcements of important Alzheimer's research are being made regularly. Caregivers should maintain a spirit of optimism and should write letters to Congress to encourage increased research funding.

WILL I GET ALZHEIMER'S DISEASE?

Alzheimer's disease can be a "familial disease," which means that some families have a particularly high incidence of the disease. Researchers believe that individuals with family members who develop Alzheimer's disease quite young, in the 40s, 50s, and 60s, may be at a greater genetic risk than people with family members developing Alzheimer's disease in their 80s and 90s. However, even having this family history does not mean that Alzheimer's disease will ever develop.

Genetic testing is available but is not considered sensitive enough to predict with precision if, or when, a person may develop the disease. Caregivers considering genetic testing should be cautious because there is no way to *prevent* Alzheimer's disease, and because test results could have a negative impact on future ability to obtain medical, life, and long-term care insurance.

The authors remember hearing a humorous but accurate rhyme that can help determine whether an individual should be concerned about his or her memory. "If you remember forgetting, that's okay; if you forget you forgot, that's not!" In other words, normal forgetfulness is a part of life. In contrast, if an individual begins telling fanciful tales to cover up forgetfulness—for example, denying that he or she ever missed a lunch date or denying that it really is his or her anniversary—serious symptoms of dementia may be occurring.

ONGOING CARE

Medical or physical problems not related to Alzheimer's disease that are left untreated can make the *person* even more confused or can produce added disabilities. Caregivers should work to reduce these so-called excess disabilities. Examples include correcting vision and hearing problems, treating pain and infection, correcting nutritional deficiencies, and reducing use of alcohol or excessive caffeine. Often, incontinence can be treated by a physician or managed with simple measures. It should not be assumed to be inevitable or untreatable. Also, the doctor or a home health agency can educate families about excellent products that can help them manage incontinence.

The *person* with Alzheimer's disease should be kept as physically active as possible with daily exercise. Alzheimer's disease is typically a slow, progressive illness. When sudden changes occur, a medical examination should be sought. For example, a *person* who suddenly begins pacing may have a fecal impaction; a *person* who becomes listless may be becoming seriously dehydrated, developing an infection, or having a reaction to medication.

Families should not be afraid to explore with the physician the use of mood-altering (psychotropic) medications to handle extreme behavior problems. Medications are not the first choice but can make an enormous difference in some situations. For example, an antidepressant medication given to a *person* with Alzheimer's disease who exhibits depression can lead to increased activity and improved quality of life.

CAREGIVING ISSUES

Alzheimer's disease affects the whole family. We cannot choose whether someone develops the disease, but we can choose how we will respond to the illness and whether it will bring our family together or drive it apart.

Caregivers cannot give what they do not have. By maintaining their own health, activities, and lives, caregivers will be able to be stronger and more supportive for the *person* with Alzheimer's disease.

Caregivers who utilize services effectively are likely to keep loved ones at home longer and are likely to stay well themselves.

CONCLUSION

These basics only scratch the surface of all the information currently available about Alzheimer's disease. The authors encourage readers to learn as much as they can about this disease, but the Best Friends model does not require extensive medical knowledge or a research background—it is conceptually easy for families and professionals to embrace. We do not have to study to learn how to become a friend.

3

Assessing Remaining Strengths and Abilities

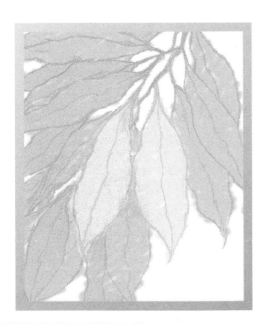

We get to know our friends very well through times spent together, conversation, and seeing them at their best and their worst. The Best Friends model teaches us that it is important to have a clear picture of the *person*. This chapter presents the Best Friends approach to assessment. A good assessment makes clear the *person's* remaining cognitive abilities and alerts us to physical problems that need attention. Equally important, a good assessment provides important information about the *person's* values, beliefs, and personality.

Why is this comprehensive assessment important? The advantage of a good assessment is that it helps us set appropriate *expectations*. For example, if an assessment reveals that the *person* with Alzheimer's disease has significant cognitive impairment, it would certainly be a disaster for him or her to try to prepare the family's income tax returns.

Expectations are important in life. We have many expectations for our friends, families, and colleagues at work. For example, we might expect one friend to be on time for every appointment or date; another friend may always run late. If we set unrealistic expectations of our tardy friend—always expecting him or her to be on time—the friendship would suffer from the continuing frustration and anger. With realistic expectations, we learn to tell our disorganized friend to meet us for the matinee at 1:00 P.M., when it really starts at 1:30 P.M.

This example reveals the benefit of setting realistic expectations. We can adjust *our* behaviors to make up for a friend's foibles. In Alzheimer's care the same holds true. Having appropriate expectations, and adjusting our interactions accordingly, can save us a world of trouble, frustration, and anger.

THE BEST FRIENDS ASSESSMENT

The Best Friends approach to conducting an assessment of the *person* with Alzheimer's disease involves striving to achieve the following goals:

1.   **To understand the state of the *person's* cognitive abilities.** A good assessment will help give us a picture of where the *person* is in terms of his or her remaining cognitive skills. It is important to consider a *person's* a) memory (short and long term), b) judgment (decisions the *person* can still make), c) speech (whether communication is easy or difficult), d) initiative (whether the *person* still has the desire to "get up and go" or initiate activities), and e) problem solving (how good is his or her ability to think through everyday problems). Finally, the assessment should look at the whole picture and ask whether the *person's* overall cognitive abilities are poor, fair, good, or excellent. What does his or her cognitive state still allow him or her to do?

2.   **To understand the current state of the *person's* physical health, including vision, hearing, and mobility.** A good assessment will remind us to keep in mind the *person's* physical strengths and weaknesses and how his or her overall physical health will affect our care plan. We cannot expect a frail older adult to enjoy a strenuous outdoor activity. This information can also help us identify problems that may appear to be related to dementia but in fact are the results of other medical conditions. Confusion, for example, might stem from very poor vision, not dementia.

3. **To reduce excess disabilities.** Regular assessments can assure that we monitor excess disabilities, the *treatable* medical problems that, left untreated, can make the symptoms of dementia worse.

4. **To understand the premorbid and postmorbid personality.** It would be impossible to be good friends with someone without really knowing his or her personality. In Alzheimer's care, we want to list the elements of a *person's* personality both before onset of the disease (premorbid) and currently (postmorbid) to help us understand what changes have occurred. When we perceive that a change is negative, such as a trusting person becoming suspicious and paranoid, we can set a goal to work on making positive changes in this area. If it provides nothing more, a personality inventory can give us a feel for how the *person* will respond to everyday situations now that he or she has Alzheimer's disease.

5. **To be able to list three things which the *person* particularly enjoys or responds to.** Family members often fall into a state of despair regarding Alzheimer's care and say that they can think of nothing that the *person* enjoys. However, some discussion and prodding almost always produces a substantial list. Perhaps the *person* enjoys or responds to making cookies, opening mail, going shopping, pressing flowers, being hugged, discussing animals, taking walks, playing a word game, or listening to music. This part of the assessment is usually just a starting point for looking at the *person's* overall care needs and potential activities.

6. **To understand who this *person* is—his or her values, beliefs, and traditions.** Caregivers should think of one or two phrases that describe the *person* before the illness. Examples could include "He believed in hard work, was a good father, and was proud of being the first in his family to get an education." Another example might be "She always enjoyed afternoon tea with friends, participated actively in her church, and was never without at least two cats in the house." We do this as part of the Best Friends assessment in order to refocus our caregiving efforts on the *person* and his or her values, concerns, and achievements.

A "DAILY TRAFFIC" CHECK

In an ideal situation, a neuropsychologist might be available to consult with a family on a monthly basis. Yet we know that most families do not get an initial neuropsychological evaluation, and those that do might get only a one-time evaluation with occasional follow-ups. Because Alzheimer's disease is progressive, it is important not to make assumptions based on an evaluation that may be out of date. The Best Friends approach to assessment is to review the overall assessment on a regular basis and make daily adjustments as needed.

Parents often give advice to their children about safely crossing intersections on their way to school, suggesting that the children take a certain route. However, good parents also stress with their children that every day is not the same. Every day the children should observe the traffic; watch the red, green, and yellow lights; and look left and right. The Best Friends approach to assessing the individual with Alzheimer's disease is to "check the daily traffic." A game plan is needed, but caregivers should be open to changing conditions. The simple assessments in this chapter should be reviewed often and expectations adjusted accordingly. After all, maybe that constantly tardy friend described earlier in this chapter has a new friend who has reformed him or her. If we continue to tell the friend to show up a half hour early for everything, he or she might be the one who becomes upset and angry!

A SIMPLE ASSESSMENT FORM

An easy-to-use form that can be used by families and professionals to make an assessment of the strengths and abilities of the *person* with Alzheimer's disease is presented on pages 33–34. The form can be used as part of an initial or continuing medical evaluation. For example, families can

1. Fax or send the *completed* form to the family doctor with a note expressing concern if a family member is exhibiting symptoms of dementia. Alerting the physician to the problem means that he or she is less likely to be fooled by the *person's* intact social graces.

2. Copy the completed form and share it with family members, particularly those who may be in denial about the *person's* illness. Alternatively, suggest that each family member complete the form and use it as the basis for a family conference.

3. Use the form on a regular basis to chart the progress of the disease and understand how the plan of care may need to be updated.

The authors encourage all families to share this form with their doctor or other health professional(s). It should, however, never replace a medical exam or neuropsychological test.

ABOUT STAGES

The Best Friends model reminds us to look at good friendship for lessons about caregiving. One such lesson is that friends do not formally assess one another constantly. Good friends are always sensing each other's daily moods, taking note of new interests, listening, and being flexible.

It is in part for this reason that the Best Friends model of care does not put people into "stages" of illness. For example, the authors have heard professionals speak of between 3 and 13 stages of Alzheimer's disease! This statement alone suggests that "stages" are not particularly helpful. The Best Friends model rejects stages for several reasons:

1. **Alzheimer's disease is a continuum of illness.** Every family will tell you that there are good days and bad days. Although there is an overall cognitive decline and eventually a physical decline, someone does not go to bed one night in "stage two" and wake up the next morning in "stage three."

2. **Stages can be misleading.** Families are either lulled into a false sense of security or overly frightened by rigid stages. For example, the authors have had family members tell us that "Mother won't wander because she's only in stage one." In fact, most individuals with Alzheimer's disease are at risk for wandering. Also, families can be scared by the invariably negative language associated with stages: for example, "This is the stage where they will lose speech, wander, burn the house down, and give away all their money."

3. **Behavior varies.** Some upsetting or difficult issues and behaviors seem to diminish as the disease progresses, while other challenges arise. It is more helpful and hopeful to focus on each individual's strengths *throughout* the disease process.

4. **Stages label people.** School systems have debated the pros and cons of labeling or tracking children, with the worry that *results*

will always match expectations. In Alzheimer's care staging people may set expectations higher or lower than they should be.

Alzheimer's care should not be standardized care.

CONCLUSION

Most assessments of individuals with Alzheimer's disease focus on their problems. The Best Friends assessment differs in that it asks us to consider what strengths and abilities remain. This shift in focus challenges caregivers, particularly professionals in day center or facility settings, to look for creative solutions.

The Best Friends model also calls for ongoing assessments. It simply will not work to assess the *person* with dementia once or twice a year. We must "check the traffic" daily and adjust our expectations of the *person* (and ourselves) accordingly.

Best Friends Assessment

1. Check the boxes that apply in order to assess the *person's* cognitive ability.

	Poor	Fair	Good	Excellent
Memory	❑	❑	❑	❑
Judgment	❑	❑	❑	❑
Language	❑	❑	❑	❑
Initiative	❑	❑	❑	❑
Problem solving	❑	❑	❑	❑
Responsiveness to instructions/requests	❑	❑	❑	❑
Overall cognitive ability	❑	❑	❑	❑

2. Check the boxes that apply in order to assess the *person*'s overall health.

	Poor	Fair	Good	Excellent
Vision	❑	❑	❑	❑
Hearing	❑	❑	❑	❑
Mobility	❑	❑	❑	❑
Overall health	❑	❑	❑	❑

3. Check the words that describe the *person's* personality before the illness and today.

Personality traits	Before illness	Today
Content	—	—
Extrovert	—	—
Fatalistic	—	—
Friendly	—	—
Happy	—	—
Introvert	—	—
Reserved	—	—
Serious	—	—
Suspicious	—	—
Timid	—	—

(continued)

List which personality traits have changed. Can you name any triggers (e.g., people, places, time of day) or theories as to why the change occurred?

Change ——————— Reason ——————————————

——————————————————————————————————

Change ——————— Reason ——————————————

——————————————————————————————————

Change ——————— Reason ——————————————

——————————————————————————————————

4. List the *person's* three most challenging behaviors:

——————————————————————————————————
——————————————————————————————————
——————————————————————————————————

Can you name any triggers (e.g., people, places, time of day) that cause these behaviors?

Problem ——————— Trigger ——————————————

——————————————————————————————————

Problem ——————— Trigger ——————————————

——————————————————————————————————

Problem ——————— Trigger ——————————————

——————————————————————————————————

5. List at least three things that the *person* seems to particularly enjoy or respond to:

——————————————————————————————————
——————————————————————————————————
——————————————————————————————————

6. List three qualities about the *person* that you would like others to know. (These qualities could include values, beliefs, traditions, or achievements.) How would the *person* have described himself or herself if asked to do so in just a few words?

——————————————————————————————————
——————————————————————————————————
——————————————————————————————————

II

The
Best
Friends
Model of
Care

*How basic rights for people with
Alzheimer's disease can lead to
improved quality of care and
quality of life, the importance of
knowing the person's life story and
incorporating it into everyday
care, and the concept of the
"knack" of care.*

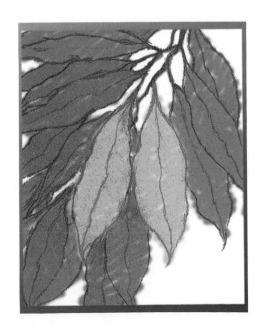

4

An Alzheimer's Disease Bill of Rights

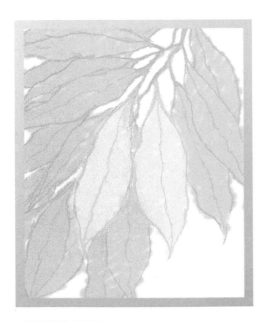

Rebecca Riley wanted to make a plan for her future. She was fortunate because her husband Jo was her greatest supporter and advocate. He argued for her when she could no longer speak for herself. What happens to people with Alzheimer's disease who are alone or have long-distance caregivers? Who speaks for them?

The authors believe the time has come for an Alzheimer's disease Bill of Rights. The Bill of Rights can serve as a touchstone for care providers for meeting client needs. The Bill of Rights can assist care providers and families when considering the ethical issues surrounding care. It can be useful to people with emerging Alzheimer's disease as they consider options and make plans. Finally, and most important, an Alzheimer's disease Bill of Rights can benefit people who cannot speak for themselves.

An Alzheimer's Disease Bill of Rights

Every *person* diagnosed with Alzheimer's disease or
   a related disorder deserves the following rights:

To be informed of one's diagnosis

To have appropriate, ongoing medical care

To be productive in work and play for as long as possible

To be treated like an adult, not like a child

To have expressed feelings taken seriously

To be free from psychotropic medications, if possible

To live in a safe, structured, and predictable environment

To enjoy meaningful activities that fill each day

To be outdoors on a regular basis

To have physical contact,
   including hugging, caressing, and hand-holding

To be with individuals who know one's life story,
   including cultural and religious traditions

To be cared for by individuals who are well trained
   in dementia care

The Best Friends Approach to Alzheimer's Care, by Virginia Bell and David Troxel.
Copyright © 1997, by Health Professions Press, Inc., Baltimore.

THE RIGHTS OF THE *PERSON* WITH ALZHEIMER'S DISEASE

Every *person* diagnosed with Alzheimer's disease or related disorders deserves the following rights. ("An Alzheimer's Disease Bill of Rights"[1] is included on page 38 to provide a handy list that can be placed in facilities, day centers, or elsewhere.)

To be informed of one's diagnosis

Typically, a patient is informed of a serious medical diagnosis, even against his or her family's wishes. For example, it is highly unusual for a physician not to inform a patient of a diagnosis of terminal cancer. When the *person* inquires, "What is wrong with me?," he or she should be told that he or she has a medical problem affecting the thinking process, memory, and judgment. If the *person* asks, "Is it Alzheimer's disease?," he or she should be told the truth. Withholding the truth and the reasons for a *person's* medical and psychological condition can be crueler than the effects of this disease.

To have appropriate, ongoing medical care

Great strides have been made in educating the public about the importance of receiving a thorough medical evaluation when symptoms of dementia appear. Some dementias are treatable. Yet, after an Alzheimer's disease diagnosis, families struggle to find appropriate, ongoing care from physicians with geriatric experience. Just as women have successfully fought for medical care that is sensitive to their special concerns and needs, we must now fight for improved geriatric care.

To be productive in work and play for as long as possible

All of us have a need to contribute to, and be a part of, the world around us—whether through work, recreation, or even helping with a simple chore. *Persons* with emerging Alzheimer's disease should be encouraged to maintain their vocational interests for as long as possible. Individuals in middle or late Alzheimer's disease benefit from meaningful activities each day.

[1] Adapted from Bell, V.M., & Troxel, D. (1994, September/October). An Alzheimer's disease bill of rights. *American Journal of Alzheimer's Care and Related Disorders & Research*, pp. 3–6; reprinted by permission.

To be treated like an adult, not like a child

The *person* has led a full life, rich in experiences. Even late into the illness, the *person* will retain a sense of his or her personal history, achievements, and values, given cues. Activities and language should be age appropriate and meaningful. A former federal judge should not be asked to cut out paper dolls. People in their 70s should not be spoken to as if they were 7 years old.

To have expressed feelings taken seriously

Care providers, family members, and others know that many individuals with dementia want to discuss their feelings and sense of loss even if they cannot always fully articulate their concerns. Family members and professionals should be willing to listen and empathize. The authors hope that the growing trend of forming support groups for individuals with emerging Alzheimer's disease will continue. They are a valuable service for the individual with dementia.

To be free from psychotropic medications, if possible

Mood-altering or psychotropic medications can be used to combat sleeplessness, anxiety, wandering, and aggression or other challenging behaviors. Although these medications can be helpful, they can also increase confusion. Most problems can be better managed by behavioral interventions or prevented altogether through improved education about the disease, better staff training in facilities, and use of the Best Friends model of care. Hugs are usually better than drugs.

To live in a safe, structured, and predictable environment

Whether it is a home or a long-term care facility, the living environment should be designed around the needs of the *person*. It should be safe and well lit, offer areas for walking or wandering, be uncluttered, and be pleasant. It should provide a structured schedule of activities and meals. Being structured and predictable does not mean boring—a rich environment that stimulates the senses (e.g., fresh flowers on the table, the smell of baking bread) can still provide the *person* with a sense of security.

To enjoy meaningful activities that fill each day

Activities should be individualized whenever possible to take into account the *person's* abilities and interests. The *person* should be given a job to do. Activities that stimulate the senses with colors, fragrances, textures, music, and the tastes of healthy foods are ideal. Exercise such as walking, dancing, ball tossing, or stretching should be part of everyday life, if possible. Above all, positive, upbeat, and life-affirming activities are encouraged.

To be outdoors on a regular basis

Individuals with dementia should have fresh air and sunshine on a regular basis. Being outdoors can also lead to enjoyable activities such as observing flowers and birds or "people watching." Just feeling warm sunshine can boost morale and stimulate the senses. Outdoor activity is particularly important for people in facilities where most activities occur indoors.

To have physical contact, including hugging, caressing, and hand-holding

Something as simple as a touch can reassure anxious individuals and bring great joy. A bear hug can distract someone about to have an outburst. If sexual intimacy is lost, hand-holding and caresses can help individuals with dementia and their loved one still feel close.

To be with individuals who know one's life story, including cultural and religious traditions

Knowing a *person's* life story and traditions enhances all aspects of Alzheimer's care. Communication is improved when caregivers can provide verbal cues. Likes and dislikes can be acknowledged. Also, appropriate activities that take into account the individual's interests and traditions can be planned. For example, it would be inappropriate to encourage someone to dance the polka if he or she belonged to a religion that prohibits dancing.

To be cared for by individuals who are well trained in dementia care

Although family caregivers should learn as much as possible about dementia care, they have the right to *demand* competent care from professionals. Reading books on dementia care, participating in support groups, and attending workshops and conferences give families and professionals more tools for providing good care and improving quality of life for the *person*.

CONCLUSION

Like the U.S. Bill of Rights, the Alzheimer's Disease Bill of Rights is not absolute. To cite a famous example from constitutional law, the right of free speech does not allow someone to yell "Fire!" in a crowded theatre when there is no fire. Likewise, the Alzheimer's Disease Bill of Rights must take into consideration each *person's* cognitive abilities and medical situation.

Yet, individuals, families, and professionals who adopt these rights will find that the result will be an improved plan of care and improved sensitivity to the *person's* needs. Facilities that adopt these rights will be informing families of their commitment to offer the highest quality of care for *persons* with dementia.

Finally, it is the authors' hope that, until a cure for Alzheimer's disease is found, these rights may give comfort to people with emerging Alzheimer's disease. They can use this bill of rights as a tool to discuss their concerns and fears and to participate as much as possible in decision making regarding their future.

5

The Art of Friendship

Spending week after week with Dicy, getting to know her, it was special. We became good friends. No—we became best friends.

—*T.J. Todd, adult day center volunteer,*

Lexington, Kentucky [1]

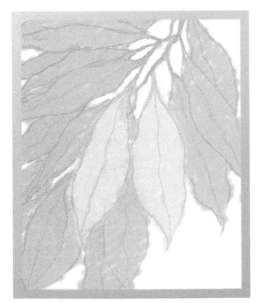

It seems that what the *person* with Alzheimer's disease really needs is a good friend. Just as many of us have friends who are always there when we need them, people with Alzheimer's disease benefit from a caregiver who says or does the right thing at the right time.

Utilizing a "best friends" approach has made the Helping Hand day program of the Lexington/Bluegrass Alzheimer's Association, founded in 1984, one of the most admired adult day center programs for people with Alzheimer's disease in the United States. At the day pro-

[1] From *Best Friends.* (1991). [Video]. (Distributed by Health Professions Press, [888] 337-8808.)

gram, well-trained volunteers provide one-on-one care for participants with Alzheimer's disease.

When the program began, the goal was to attract enough volunteers to have individualized care. Because the program started out
small and had strong community support, it achieved this goal. Volunteers found the work rewarding, and in 1995 an extraordinary 148
volunteers were active in the program, including many who had
volunteered for over 10 years.

As the authors began developing this model of Alzheimer's care,
we continually recalled the success of Helping Hand and other adult
day programs we had visited throughout the United States. Staff and
volunteers at these programs were providing a level of care that surprised many professionals. The participants with dementia were thriv-
ing, as were the volunteers. How could this success be explained?

We soon realized that these centers represented friendship at its
best. The relationships among staff, volunteers, and participants exemplified the art of good friendship. We found an abundance of
commitment, give and take, and humor. People seemed to want to be
with each other. These insights led us to the view that there is a strong
relationship between good friendship and the best Alzheimer's care.
Indeed, the qualities of good friendship contain lessons about Alzheimer's care that form the building blocks for the Best Friends model.

"Elements of Friendship and Alzheimer's Care" (see pp. 46–47)
lists the qualities of friendship and how they relate to Alzheimer's
care. These qualities are described individually in this chapter.

FRIENDS KNOW EACH OTHER'S
HISTORY AND PERSONALITY

Typically, people become friends because they have something in
common; perhaps they graduated from the same high school or college or both enjoy Saturday night bowling. As the friendship grows,
they learn more about each other—how many brothers and sisters
each has, their birthdays and birthplaces, cultural and religious
traditions, hobbies, and special achievements. As much as we think
we know about our friends, there are often surprises. Perhaps it turns
out a friend once thought to be strictly a country music fan has a
passion for opera.

Friends also become good judges of each other's moods and

personalities. A friend develops a sense of timing—where and when not to tease someone. Friends even begin to understand each other's problem-solving style, knowing when a word of advice is welcome and when it may be resented.

Friendship in Alzheimer's Care

A Best Friend Becomes the *Person's* Memory

It is often difficult to learn biographical information from the *person*. He or she may have forgotten much of the past, or simply be unable to recall the names of people, places, or things in his or her life. A Best Friend should learn as much as possible about the *person* (see Chapter 6 for an expanded explanation of this point) in order to offer cues and reminders of his or her previous achievements.

Judge Jean Auxier was a well-respected U.S. Attorney for the Eastern District of Kentucky. After he became ill with Alzheimer's disease, he rarely spoke. Yet he glowed when reminded of his achievements, and he laughed loudly when an old friend facetiously said, "You know, Judge, I never have forgiven you for sentencing me to 5 to 10."

The judge's visitor said just the right thing.

Howard Shipps, a retired seminary professor, came to the adult day center every day dressed in coat and tie, ready for work. He beamed when reminded of his past success as a teacher, and when introduced as a distinguished professor church history, he smiled and said, "Yes, and much more!"

Howard would have sat quietly, uninvolved, if he had not been reminded of his past.

A Best Friend Is Sensitive to the *Person's* Traditions

Even late in the illness, the *person* often retains his or her values and traditions.

Joe Blackhurst speaks often of his childhood in Scotland. One day, a volunteer who had just gotten back from a trip to Scotland came to the adult day program with souvenirs, and even wore a kilt to show the group. She expected Joe to be thrilled with her stories. However, remembering his childhood, he frowned and said that (in his time) a woman would never wear a kilt! He was remembering correctly. When Joe lived in Scotland, women never wore kilts.

ELEMENTS OF FRIENDSHIP

Friends Know Each Other's History and Personality
In Alzheimer's care, a Best Friend
  Becomes the *person's* memory
  Is sensitive to the *person's* traditions
  Learns the *person's* personality, moods, and
    problem-solving style

Friends Do Things Together
In Alzheimer's care, a Best Friend
  Involves the *person* in daily activities and chores
  Initiates activities
  Ties activities into the *person's* past skills and interests
  Encourages the *person* to enjoy the simpler things in life
  Remembers to celebrate special occasions

Friends Communicate
In Alzheimer's care, a Best Friend
  Listens skillfully
  Speaks skillfully
  Asks questions skillfully
  Speaks using body language
  Gently encourages participation in conversations

Friends Build Self-Esteem
In Alzheimer's care, a Best Friend
  Gives compliments often
  Carefully asks for advice or opinions
  Always offers encouragement
  Offers congratulations

and Alzheimer's Care

Friends Laugh Often
In Alzheimer's care, a Best Friend
    Tells jokes and funny stories
    Takes advantage of spontaneous fun
    Uses self-deprecating humor often

Friends Are Equals
In Alzheimer's care, a Best Friend
    Does not talk down to the *person*
    Always works to protect the dignity of the *person,*
        to "save face"
    Does not assume a supervisory role
    Recognizes that learning is a two-way street

Friends Work at the Relationship
In Alzheimer's care, a Best Friend
    Is not overly sensitive
    Does more than 50% of the work
    Builds a trusting relationship
    Shows affection often

The Best Friends Approach to Alzheimer's Care, by Virginia Bell and David Troxel.
Copyright © 1997, by Health Professions Press, Inc., Baltimore.

Joe Blackhurst is proud of his heritage and loves being reminded that he is a Scot.

Leota Kilkenny always enjoyed lunch at the day center (located in a church building). One day, she refused to eat, saying, "I cannot. I must not now." After several attempts to encourage her to eat failed, she began to get agitated. Staff let her skip the meal. Later, her daughter Ann solved the mystery by saying that, while they were driving to the day center, she told her mother that they were going to the program "at the Church." Ann told the staff, "Mother is Catholic and must have thought she was going to her church and would be taking communion. In her tradition, you do not eat within an hour before receiving communion."

This is an example of how a deeply felt tradition, even one that cannot be expressed in words, can affect daily care.

A Best Friend Learns the *Person's* Personality, Moods, and Problem-Solving Style

Personalities and problem-solving styles do sometimes change with the onset of Alzheimer's disease, but more often than not the underlying attitudes and styles remain. For example, a *person* who always coped well with adversity may bring some of this resiliency into Alzheimer's disease. A *person* who has always been a "take-charge" individual or in positions of authority often will not take kindly to being told what to do.

Marydean Evans always told her friends and family that she was not a morning person and could be in a bad mood until mid-morning. Staff and volunteers empathized and would always greet her with a remark such as, "Marydean, I know you're not a morning person. Would some coffee help? How about five cups?"

Knowing Marydean's quirk, staff would never press her to be involved too early in the morning, respecting her desire to wake up slowly over some hot coffee.

FRIENDS DO THINGS TOGETHER

Many friendships start at the workplace, church, or school. People will meet, discover common interests, and build a friendship based on doing things together. Friends enjoy all sorts of activities, including going to movies, taking walks, playing sports, taking a trip or vacation, working on a volunteer project, doing crafts, going shopping, or simply talking on the phone.

Activities can be planned in advance but are often spontaneous. Good friends find that simple activities such as renting a video or going to the grocery store together can give as much pleasure as an elaborately planned outing.

Friendship in Alzheimer's Care

A Best Friend Involves the *Person* in Activities and Chores

The *person* with Alzheimer's disease and a Best Friend can do a project together, such as cleaning the kitchen. Even with limited skills, the *person* can often help with daily chores, such as drying the dishes or stacking the newspapers to recycle. The key to all of these activities is to get the person involved, to encourage him or her to be a part of life.

Edna Carroll Greenwade led a busy life as a homemaker and as a buyer for Francis' Department Store in Prestonsburg, Kentucky. When nothing was going on, Edna Carroll remembered that "Idle hands are the devil's workshop." She was happiest when she watered plants, stacked chairs, or polished the piano.

The key to successfully working with Edna Carroll was to remember she loved to stay busy.

The Gajardos were together at home for 10 years after Sergio ("Serge"), an executive for a large company, was diagnosed with Alzheimer's disease. Little by little, many things they once enjoyed were no longer possible. Yet, his wife, Gertrude, found that he could still enjoy many daily chores, such as chopping up vegetables for a stir-fry dinner they could then enjoy.

Serge felt competent and successful when he helped to prepare the evening meal.

A Best Friend Initiates Activities

Because the *person* often loses the ability to initiate activities, it is a mistake to always ask the *person* if he or she wants to do something. The answer will often be "No." Instead, a Best Friend could say, for example, "I would like to take a walk. Come on, join me! It's great to exercise with you."

The Matsumura family of Carpinteria, California, worked together to provide care to their father, "Mas," diagnosed with Alzheimer's disease in his early 50s. The family became involved in the Santa Barbara Alzheimer's Association fund-raising Memory Walk, and told Mas that he was needed that day. Before the walk started, Mas helped put up tables. The family gave him encouragement and supervised help. Afterward, he spoke about how much fun he had and how useful he felt.

Participating in an important activity with his family made Mas feel a part of life.

Marian Witte's daughter Claralee planned time each day to play the piano and sing with her mother, an activity they both enjoyed. Marian liked to be reminded of her childhood when the family would gather most evenings, sit or stand around the piano, and sing.

Marian could not initiate this activity, but once the music began she participated enthusiastically.

A Best Friend Ties Activities into the *Person's* Past Skills and Interests

The Best Friend can use the *person's* life story to identify old skills that can be tapped into.

Beverly Wheeler[2] is proud of her achievements as a kindergarten and elementary schoolteacher. Despite her diagnosis of early Alzheimer's disease, she wants to continue helping others. Her husband, Michael, encourages her to make occasional visits to classes and to attend conferences to speak about her experience with Alzheimer's disease. By continuing to teach, Beverly feels that she is making a contribution to the people around her.

After the day center staff learned that Tennie Clayton had a lifelong interest in quilting, they asked her daughter Gretchen to bring in an example of her work. With a big smile, Tennie arrived the next day with a quilt she was "piecing" together. Everyone complimented her on the work with comments such as, "What beautiful colors!" and "Look at those small stitches!" Tennie was elated.

Because people have led such full, rich lives, the possibilities for activities linked to the past are unlimited.

---

[2] Beverly Wheeler tells her story in the video *My Challenge with Alzheimer's Disease,* © 1996 Philogenesis Productions and Friendship Center. (Distributed by Terra Nova Films, 9848 S. Winchester Avenue, Chicago, IL 60643.)

A Best Friend Encourages
the *Person* to Enjoy the Simple Things in Life

Simple things are often the best things in Alzheimer's care. For example, it can be pleasurable for both the *person* and the Best Friend to walk in a shopping mall. The Best Friend can comment, "That teenager over there has green hair!" or "Look at that triple-scoop ice-cream cone! Do you think you could eat all of that?"

Serge Gajardo and his wife found pleasure in a simple activity; they often stopped by garage sales. Serge had collected wood carvings and art from all over the world, and he still enjoyed browsing for treasures and irresistible bargains.

Silence is also part of any friendship. Sometimes it is nice to simply sit in a comfortable chair and watch the world go by, or be in a room and watch friends or family play a game or watch television. The *person* can still feel a sense of involvement and security by being in the presence of others.

A Best Friend Remembers to Celebrate Special Occasions

The ritual of a birthday party, anniversary celebration, Veteran's Day parade, or other long-held traditions can bring back many positive memories for the *person*. Special occasions can be celebrated throughout the year, making a big day out of a birthday or other family event.

Elaine Schratwieser and Rodger Currie got married twice, once in a church and again 7 weeks later in a renewal of their vows at her mother's adult day center. The second wedding was complete with wedding cake, photographers, music, and a priest. Not only was it an enormous pleasure for her mother to "host" the event at her day center but the other participants enormously enjoyed the event; a wedding had deep symbolic meaning to which all could relate.

FRIENDS COMMUNICATE

The best friendships often involve a lot of talking. Whether it is on the telephone or over the office water cooler, friends generally love to swap stories, gossip, share ideas, and confide in one another. Friends are also there to listen to each other, in good and bad times.

Friendship in Alzheimer's Care

A Best Friend Listens Skillfully

In Alzheimer's care, it is important to try to be there for the *person* when he or she wants to talk about his or her feelings. *Persons* should be given time to offer their feelings or ideas. Sometimes patience is rewarded with an insight.

When Thelma Moody is feeling frightened or angry, her husband, Julian, has learned to sit quietly with her, hold her gently, listen to the language of her emotions, and respond to her emotional needs.

Communication can come from the heart as well as from the head.

Betty Justice seldom made much sense with her parade of words, but day center staff were used to "reading" her face and responding. One day, while trying to speak, she said with some force, "He's sick." Trained to listen carefully, staff were surprised by this clear message and responded, "I'm so sorry." Later that day, staff found out that her husband was in the hospital.

By listening carefully to a *person*, even when he or she cannot be readily understood, it is often possible to get a clear message when least expected.

A Best Friend Speaks Skillfully

The *person* should be given every opportunity to understand what is being said. A Best Friend should use short, simple, direct sentences with descriptive language, such as, "Please hand me my red purse," instead of "Hand me that thing." Also, we must remember to speak clearly, slowly, and loudly if the *person* has a hearing impairment.

Knowing the person's life story is very important in skillful communication.

Edna Edwards loves to converse but has major difficulty finding the right words. When her Best Friend supplies familiar words, saying, "Those kids at Picadome school were lucky to have you as a teacher!," Edna can respond, "Picadome, that's my school! Those little ones, I miss them." Conversation can continue about early childhood days, her teaching, and her school-children, all because her Best Friend knew some familiar names of people, places, and things in Edna's life.

A Best Friend Asks Questions Skillfully

The *person* may become easily frustrated if asked questions to which he or she does not know the answer.

When Evelyn Talbott, a retired librarian, returned from a trip to the beach, a friend asked skillful questions about the trip. She did not ask, "Where did you go?" or "What did you do?" Instead, she asked, "Did you and your husband, Bob, have a good time watching those big waves on the ocean?" The cues of "husband," "Bob," "big waves," and "ocean" allowed Evelyn to answer, "Yes, and they were big ones!" She and her friend could continue to reminisce about their times at the beach.

Open-ended questions such as "What do you do for fun?" are also appropriate because there are no right or wrong answers.

A Best Friend Speaks Using Body Language

Because verbal skills are diminished, body language becomes very important in Alzheimer's care. A Best Friend should greet the *person* warmly, smile broadly, and hold out a hand. The handshake still holds special meaning with older people, who remember a time when everyone in polite company would shake hands. Almost always, the *person* will respond with a handshake. A mutual handshake is the beginning of a bond, a deep-rooted symbol that one is a friend, not a foe. Eye contact is also important. A Best Friend should try to look directly at the *person* and "catch" his or her eye. The *person* will be better able to focus on what is being communicated and the Best Friend will be able to "read" the *person's* face, to judge his or her reaction to the words.

In Alzheimer's care, talking with the hands is encouraged. Gestures such as tapping the seat on a chair can help the *person* get the message to sit down.

Because of Mary Burmaster's hearing loss, body language is especially effective for a day center volunteer relating to her. After making eye contact, the volunteer would say, "Mary, lunch is ready." The volunteer would then touch her gently on the shoulder, pat her hand, and guide her to the table.

The volunteer's gentle touch spoke volumes.

A Best Friend Gently
Encourages Participation in Conversations

It is important to include the *person* in everyday conversation as much as possible. A Best Friend can ask open-ended questions such as "Tell me about . . . ?" or "What do you think about . . . ?"

Carmen K. Singh cared for her father, Marcus P. Powell, a former University of Iowa professor. After he had lost much of his ability to initiate conversation, he was encouraged by his daughter to speak. She would ask questions such as, "What do you think about wearing this bow tie today?" or "Could you tell me about that fishing pole you had as a kid?"

FRIENDS BUILD SELF-ESTEEM

A good friendship brings out the best in each *person* and builds self-esteem. It involves a mutual support system, giving each other constructive criticism and feedback and, when the chips are down, giving unconditional support. Friends look at strengths more than weaknesses.

Friendship in Alzheimer's Care
A Best Friend Gives Compliments Often

Telling a *person* "You look nice today" or "You really did a good job gardening" builds self-esteem. A compliment also can "disarm" the *person* who is having a bad day or bad moment. The compliment distracts the *person*, moving him or her away from the problem or concern. Compliments inevitably evoke a smile.

"Mas" Matsumura loves to bowl and would do it almost every day if his family agreed. During one trip to the bowling alley, Mas was very rusty. After a few gutter balls, his family complimented him on his past skills by saying, "Dad, you're a great bowler. Try again." Mas went on to bowl several strikes.

Mas smiled broadly as his family cheered his success.

When Marcus P. Powell's family sensed that he was feeling sad, his children and grandchildren would often compliment him on his past successes. "Papa," they would say, "you can be so proud of all those students you helped in Iowa. You still have a lot of things to teach all of us."

A Best Friend Carefully Asks for Advice or Opinions

Another way to show a *person* that he or she is valued is by asking him or her for an opinion. The question need not be about the national debt or foreign trade. Instead, a man could ask, "I didn't have a chance to look in the mirror today. Do you think my tie matches my shirt?" This could lead to a lengthy discussion about fabrics, textures, colors, changing widths of ties, and perhaps even a new wardrobe.

Christine Clark was a traditional homemaker who had cooked since she was a teenager. She loved it when volunteers in the day program would ask her for advice about what to cook for dinner. Volunteers could also ask her opinions related to the meal: "Christine, do you think mashed potatoes or rice go better with fried chicken? Which would you cook?"

A Best Friend Always Offers Encouragement

Persons with Alzheimer's disease need as much encouragement as possible, which can take many forms. Sometimes it is valuable to encourage the *person* by reminding him or her of his or her value as a friend: "You add so much to my life" or "We're just like sisters." The *person* can also be encouraged to attempt a particular task, especially a task that seems possible to accomplish. A Best Friend might say, "I could use your help in putting this puzzle together. Would you come sit by me and help out?"

A beautiful scarf, creatively displayed to complement her outfit, was Edna Carroll Greenwade's hallmark. One day, the director of the day center brought a collection of scarves and encouraged Edna Carroll to show everyone how to wear them. Edna beamed as she helped each participant arrange her scarf and, as the fashion show of scarves passed by her for inspection, she exclaimed, "I'm so glad to be of help!"

Often, gentle encouragement is all that is needed to practice an old skill.

A Best Friend Offers Congratulations

In Alzheimer's care, the *person* should be congratulated often for small and big successes.

When Edna Edwards's granddaughter was a finalist in the Miss Kentucky beauty pageant, Helping Hand volunteers "congratulated" Edna often for her successful granddaughter: "Edna, congratulations on your granddaugh-

ter's success; Mary Dudley must have gotten her good looks from you!"
Edna would often respond, "You know it!"

A *person* can also be congratulated for a success in his or her past.

Pauline Huffman was the first woman in Lexington, Kentucky, to ever bowl a sanctioned "perfect" 300 game. For this accomplishment, she was inducted into the Lexington Bowling Association's Hall of Fame. She also once made a hole-in-one in golf. Pauline loved to be reminded of these successes. She did not always remember the details of the actual event but seemed to remember well the emotions and good feelings associated with that championship game and that hole-in-one.

Congratulating a *person* can make him or her feel accomplished and proud.

FRIENDS LAUGH OFTEN

Humor is a powerful element in all relationships. Humor helps people enjoy shared experiences, relieves tension, and brings people together. Many researchers have also confirmed that laughter has positive physiological effects, boosting the immune system and lowering blood pressure.

Friendship in Alzheimer's Care
A Best Friend Tells Jokes and Funny Stories

Even the corniest old joke can evoke big laughs from someone with dementia. Funny stories are also popular, particularly ones involving either the caregiver or the *person*. For example, a Best Friend might say, "I still haven't forgiven you for eating the last piece of grandmother's pie that fourth of July."

We should not forget that the *person* can sometimes remember or tell a great story or joke.

In spite of the fact that he had had a series of strokes, Jerry Ruttenberg retained his great sense of humor. When a volunteer in the day center handed him corn on the cob, he said loudly, "Oh, shucks." Another time, in answer to the serious question, "How do sand dollars reproduce?," he quipped, "They give birth to baby dimes."

It can almost be a running joke in some friendships: "Not that story again, I've heard it before!" Yet in Alzheimer's care, a story that is repeated often can be a favorite with the *person*. It may be that they are simply not remembering hearing it before. More likely, they connect with the smiles, laughter, and joy associated with the story.

A Best Friend Takes Advantage of Spontaneous Fun

Things happen spontaneously that are often humorous for the *person* and the people around him or her. Laughter can come from watching staff at a nursing facility chase a pet rabbit that has gotten free from its cage.

Gary Dewhirst, a program director of an adult day center in San Luis Obispo, California, announced to the group with great fanfare that he was personally going to barbecue a turkey for the Thanksgiving luncheon. He set up the barbecue on the patio, and the group watched the preparations. All was going well until the turkey caught fire. Gary had to use a fire extinguisher to douse the flames, ruining the turkey. After the initial shock, a call was made to Domino's (pizza). Everyone teased Gary later that only he could provide the group with "traditional" Thanksgiving pizza.

A Best Friend Uses Self-Deprecating Humor Often

Friends are not afraid to be the butt of their own jokes. Embarrassing moments happen to all of us, but are a particular concern of people with Alzheimer's disease. When a *person* forgets a name of an old friend, a good response from a Best Friend could be "That's okay, I'm glad I'm not the only one who forgets things" or "I looked all over for my glasses last week and then found them—right on my nose." What self-deprecating humor does is reassure the *person* that he or she is not the only one in the world who can be forgetful. It also diffuses negative situations, and helps the *person* stay in a positive mood. A good self-deprecating remark also allows for laughter to break the tension, for a frown to turn into a smile.

The spotlight at the day center was on Marydean Evans as she demonstrated the steps to the waltz. The group was enjoying the occasion when suddenly Marydean began looking for something to show the group. She was sure that she had it when she came to the program that morning: "I'm always losing my things and I wanted to show it to everyone." In keeping with the celebratory mood, her Best Friend quipped, "I have the same problem sometimes. Good thing my head is securely fastened. I'd lose it too!"

FRIENDS ARE EQUALS

No friendship will survive condescending behavior. Everyone has different strengths and weaknesses, but differences should be celebrated rather than dwelled on.

Friendship in Alzheimer's Care

A Best Friend Does Not Talk Down to the *Person*

Condescending language is never appropriate in good Alzheimer's care. Examples of inappropriate language include speaking in an exaggerated, slow, and measured voice when not necessary; being insensitive; using childlike language; being flippant; not giving the *person* time to respond to a question; asking inappropriate and embarrassing questions; or "talking through" a person as though he or she was not present.

Rubena Dean enjoyed looking at cards that contained brief biographies of famous women. One day she was trying to recall facts about Helen Keller when she lost her train of thought. A sensitive friend felt her pain at not being able to finish and simply said, "I'm sorry." Her friend did not condescend by trying to negate or dismiss her feelings. Rubena needed her friend to identify with her pain.

A Best Friend Always Works to Protect the Dignity of the *Person,* to "Save Face"

Many people with Alzheimer's disease remain fiercely proud.

When Margaret Brubaker's friends or family visited, they were often concerned that she was not eating well. She was very proud and refused gifts of food, saying that she was not hungry or had "just eaten an enormous meal!" A volunteer took a different approach. During one visit, he said, "Margaret, you could do me such a favor. Bananas were on sale this week and I bought 3 pounds. My wife went to the store separately and she bought 3 pounds. We just don't know what to do with all these bananas. It would help us so much if you'd take some off our hands."

Margaret took the bananas with delight because she was doing her friend a favor.

Another example of saving face is letting the *person* off the hook if he or she fails. If someone asks an awkward question ("How many children do you have?") and a Best Friend can see the *person* struggling, he or she can jump in and provide an answer, change the subject, or tell a self-deprecating joke so that the *person* will not feel humiliated.

A Best Friend Does Not Assume a Supervisory Role

No bosses or employees should exist in Alzheimer's care. Friends are equals, and the *person* often responds negatively if he or she has a feeling of being bossed around.

Helen King, a retired librarian, was diagnosed with early Alzheimer's disease. She enjoys being "in charge" of the adult day center's library. Helen often comments about the day center program: "I enjoy it so much because there are no bosses here."

Using finesse (see p. 93) can help caregivers avoid becoming the "bad guy" by shifting responsibility to others. A son can say, "Dad, I know you want to keep driving, but the motor vehicle department says no." This is better for his relationship with his father than saying, "Dad, I don't think you should be driving."

A Best Friend Recognizes that Learning Is a Two-Way Street

Equality means learning things from each other. Many volunteers who work in adult day centers or long-term care facilities comment that they learn much from the people they care about. Many people with dementia can still share stories from their personal histories, express compassion and concern, or demonstrate old skills and hobbies.

Dicy Jenkins was a walking encyclopedia of information about plants and herbs used for health and healing. She knew how to use juniper berries, ginseng, feverfew, bee pollen, and burdock root for medicinal purposes. Volunteers at the adult day center often took copious notes on Dicy's remedies to relieve their ailments.

FRIENDS WORK AT THE RELATIONSHIP

Every friendship has its difficult moments. Something said is miscon-strued, or a friend disappoints us in some fashion. Clearly no friend-ship will survive a continuing series of disappointments, but best friends discuss disagreements and work them out. Good friendships can handle some rough-and-tumble moments, constructive teasing, and high spirits. Good friendships also require work and commitment. Friends need to stay in touch by phone or letter, and initiate activities with each other.

Friendship in Alzheimer's Care

A Best Friend Is Not Overly Sensitive

Friends must recognize that problems, when they occur, are normally part of the disease process, not part of the *person*. Sometimes, inhibitions are reduced by dementia. The *person* may say some surprising things.

Geri Greenway valued great art, music, stylish clothes, and beautiful jewelry. When a volunteer in the day center program asked Geri what she thought of some new costume jewelry she had brought to the day program to display, Geri replied, "Well, it looks like a bunch of junk to me." The experience of the volunteer showed. She replied to the group humorously, "Ask a question, get an answer."

A Best Friend Does More than 50% of the Work

In Alzheimer's care, clearly most of the work is done by the friend without dementia. Just as we would give a friend having tough times some latitude, we should do the same or more with the *person* with Alzheimer's disease.

Howard Woods amazed his friends and family with his daily care of his wife, Emma, who had late Alzheimer's disease. He told friends that they had not really had the best marriage, often having disagreements. Yet he said that, through his time with her, caring about her, and doing things for her that he never could imagine doing for anyone, he had fallen in love with her all over again.

A Best Friend Builds a Trusting Relationship

Building a trusting relationship takes work. The concept of "caregiving integrity" is examined in Chapter 7, and it is an important part of the Best Friends model. Trust can be gained when caregivers demonstrate confident, consistent, loving care. Obviously there are times when problems occur, and some individuals with Alzheimer's disease are distrustful of the world. Piece by piece, however, a trusting relationship can be built.

Helen King was very distrustful of the concept of an adult day center when she first attended one. She is very aware of her memory loss and did not want to expose her limitations. As she became familiar with the program volunteers, she realized that they were very supportive and respectful of her remaining abilities. Gradually, her trust grew, and she now speaks enthusiastically about attending her "class" each day.

A Best Friend Shows Affection Often

The authors know of some long-term care facilities and adult day centers that have a "three hugs a day" rule. Best Friends show the *person* with Alzheimer's disease affection as often as possible in various ways, including compliments, holding hands, a pat on the back, hugs (why not three hugs an hour?), and smiles.

During a program on South America, a staff member asked for a volunteer to help her demonstrate a typical South American greeting. Serge Gajardo anticipated some fun and volunteered. When he was kissed, first on one cheek and then on the other, he was quick to say, "Let's keep this good stuff going!"

RECASTING RELATIONSHIPS

A Word for Family Caregivers

A major challenge for families coping with Alzheimer's disease is that memories fade and identities change. A mother, father, sister, brother, husband, wife, or partner may no longer know us or understand his or her relationship to us. Many despair of this loss. A woman's mother may have always been her closest confidante and strongest supporter. Now, she does not know her daughter. A husband who always remembered every birthday and anniversary may no longer understand that the woman caring for him is his wife.

As difficult as it seems, family caregivers coping with Alzheimer's disease often are forced to recast their relationships with loved ones. The authors recommend that, rather than stay in a state of despair, caregivers work through the pain and focus on gaining maximum value from the present. Family members should think of their loved one now as a friend, a *best friend*. Recasting this relationship does not mean taking away love, or loving him or her any less— the *person* is still family. It simply means approaching *the relationship* differently.

By treating a loved one as a friend, utilizing the ideas and approaches described in this chapter, family members will find that the pain and loss they are experiencing will diminish. In good friendship, there is joy, and we all know that sometimes relationships with friends are easier and less emotionally complex than family relationships.

One caregiver told us that he had always had a troublesome relationship with his father—so bad, in fact, that he ran away from home at age 16. He now cares for his father full time and says they've never been closer. They take a daily walk together, have an evening scotch and soda, and watch the grandchildren play soccer. They have found that they now enjoy each other's company. Because the father has forgotten much of the past and is often unsure of his relationship with his son, the son has realized that he, too, must let go of past slights and injustices. "What's the point of me dwelling on it?" the caregiver asks. "What's past is past."

Like many caregivers, the son never dreamed he would be in the position of taking care of his father, a father whom he admits disliking for much of his life. However, caregivers do what they have to do. This family's approach to Alzheimer's care has helped heal not only the son's relationship with his father but also wounds he has carried inside himself.

When family caregivers recast their relationships, there will be several benefits, as follows:

- Take advantage of the principles of friendship to gain new ideas for handling day-to-day care in a more natural, positive way.

- Prevent problems before they happen.

- Form a new relationship with a loved one based on getting the most out of every day.

- Replace the stress and strain of caregiving with satisfaction.

A Word to Professional Caregivers

The authors recognize that the job descriptions of paid staff in nursing facilities, adult day centers, or other settings who work with individuals with Alzheimer's disease usually do not include "Be a friend to your resident." However, the Best Friends model will pay many dividends if staff treat residents or day center participants as they would a best friend. The model will allow staff to do the following:

1. Approach individuals with Alzheimer's disease as they would a good friend, demonstrating that they are respected and valued.

The *person* will respond to the positive feelings he or she receives from staff.

2. Learn tools to use in any situation to improve behavior, prevent problems, and make the job easier. Staff will learn better ways of communicating, doing activities, and working with people with dementia. It is always better to prevent difficult behavior than it is to deal with it when it happens.

3. Easily train other staff members with varying educational backgrounds, divergent languages and cultural backgrounds, and different experiences.

4. Improve morale through the introduction of an upbeat and life-affirming model. Facilities and centers adopting the Best Friends approach will find that staff morale is improved and that volunteer recruitment efforts are enhanced.

CONCLUSION

Adopting the Best Friends model will provide many benefits to both the *person* and the caregiver. As this chapter has demonstrated, many elements of good friendship can be applied to Alzheimer's care. The lessons are simple to understand and simple to put into practice.

Alzheimer's care can be challenging. By adopting the common-sense strategies contained in the Best Friends model and recasting relationships, caregivers can become better prepared to cope with the challenges.

6

The
Life
Story

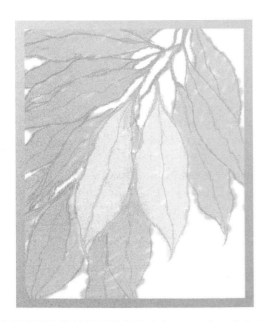

How well do we know our friends? Even if they are acquaintances or casual friends, we can usually describe their occupations, marital status, general interests, favorite foods, type of car, hobbies, and other details. What about our *closest* friends? We usually know much more about them, including defining childhood experiences, family traditions, even closely held secrets. We also know their strengths and weaknesses and understand their basic personalities.

In creating the Best Friends model of Alzheimer's care, it occurred to the authors that the average nursing facility staff member, adult day center staff member, or other professional/paid caregiver has only limited knowledge of his or her residents or clients. For example, facilities take biographical information from new residents, but often the information is rather cursory and may or may not be learned by all staff involved in a resident's care. This brief biography works well when the individuals can fill in the missing pieces, sharing their life stories with all who want to listen.

However, Alzheimer's care is different. People with Alzheimer's disease cannot tell their stories. They may not remember their family names and backgrounds, jobs, marital status, and children. They may offer conflicting information or mix up their own history with that of other relatives.

A *written* life story gathered from family, friends, and even the *person* is a critical part of the Best Friends model of care. We must

- Learn details of the *person's* past in order to improve communication, enjoy successful activities, provide necessary cues, and get in touch with distant memories
- Be able to tell familiar stories and paint a picture of past achievements
- Honor traditions, including religious values

Because *persons* with dementia can no longer write their autobiographies, we must become their biographers.

In effect, the Best Friends model makes a simple proposal: In Alzheimer's care, we cannot be only acquaintances; to bring out the best in people with Alzheimer's disease, we need to know them as well as we know our *best friends.*

This chapter examines how to collect the *person's* life story and incorporate it into daily situations. Care providers can think of themselves as detectives. Collecting and recording information to write a good life story can involve solving family mysteries, interviewing distant relatives and friends, reviewing old photographs and clippings, and asking the *person* him- or herself for information, if possible.

This chapter begins with an outline of the key elements to be included in the life story, along with some meaningful anecdotes about individuals and families who have faced Alzheimer's disease. The reader will learn that the life story can be woven into all aspects of Alzheimer's care. The chapter ends with an expanded life story of Rebecca Matheny Riley, including notations on the ways it can be used to provide outstanding care to and meaningful activities for other people with Alzheimer's disease.

INGREDIENTS OF THE LIFE STORY

This section outlines the ingredients that help create a comprehensive written life story of someone with Alzheimer's disease (see the form "Recipe for the Life Story" on p. 68). Just as recipes differ, we can choose the important information to include in the life story, or stories, that we write.

Childhood

In Alzheimer's care, understanding the *person's* earliest years is sometimes more important than familiarity with the later years. Because many people with dementia recall childhood, we want to know as much as possible about this influential time.

We can begin by asking what was the date and where was the place of birth. However, we want to do more than simply record the basics. We want to get a feel for the *atmosphere* in which the *person* was raised. Was the birthplace rural or urban? Was the *person* raised in a coal camp in Appalachia or in a Park Avenue penthouse? Did the *person* raise chickens or buy them? What were the main industries of the town in which the *person* was raised? Did his or her hometown have any special claim to fame? Someone might remember his or her birthplace as the place where the first Model A Ford came off the assembly line, where Corningware was invented, or where everyone looked at the Eiffel Tower as the city's center. For example, a friend of the authors who lives in Stockbridge, Massachusetts, notes with pride that it is the hometown of Norman Rockwell and that members of her family appear in his paintings. When available, this information can be a fascinating part of the life story.

We should try to piece together even a simple family tree of the *person's* childhood, with the names of his or her grandparents, parents, and siblings. We should ask whether there were any particularly influential relatives, such as an adored older sister or a grandmother who baked prize-winning apple pies. We must learn more about these key relatives, if possible. For example, at one adult day center, staff were amazed to learn that 3 of the 15 participants in that day's program had an identical twin.

Does the *person* remember his or her first day of school? This is usually a milestone. Was it a one-room schoolhouse or a large school? Was school enjoyable? Was the *person* a good student? Was there a favorite subject or favorite teacher? The authors remember one woman who took pride in remembering that she was "Miss Seventh-Grade Square Root."

We should be sure to discover if the *person's* parents had an unusual (at least as compared to the present) occupation. Did they

RECIPE FOR THE LIFE STORY

The authors recommend the following ingredients to make a comprehensive life story. The ingredients are listed in chronological order for convenience, but the events are not necessarily limited to those years. For example, someone may have been in military service throughout his or her working life.

Childhood
Birthdate and birthplace
Parents and grandparents
Brothers and sisters
Early education
Pets

Adolescence
Name of high school
Favorite classes
Friends and interests
Hobbies and sports
First job

Young adulthood
College and work
Marriage(s)/relationship(s)
Family
Clubs and/or community
    involvement
First home
Military service

Middle age
Grandchildren
Hobbies
Work/family role
Clubs and organizations
Community involvement

Later years
Life achievements and
    accomplishments
Hobbies
Travel
Family

Other major ingredients
Ethnicity
Religious background
Awards
Special skills

The Best Friends Approach to Alzheimer's Care, by Virginia Bell and David Troxel.
Copyright © 1997, by Health Professions Press, Inc., Baltimore.

deliver milk or pilot the local riverboat? Many older people today emigrated or were children of immigrants. It is often meaningful to find out the country from which the family emigrated and how the family found its way to the United States. Sometimes these stories involve high drama—life-threatening escapes from an oppressed country, a difficult voyage on an unsafe boat, or travel to the Oklahoma Territory in a covered wagon.

We should also learn about any life-defining childhood events. We certainly hope to find happy childhood experiences, but we want to understand any traumas in order to avoid triggering unhappy memories. Perhaps a defining moment was winning a student-of-the-year award or a statewide fishing contest. Maybe it was the day the *person's* father was elected to the state legislature. It can be valuable to know whether an individual had a troubled childhood (e.g., being orphaned at an early age, surviving a wartime childhood). Also important are childhood traumas, perhaps the death of a close friend or a natural disaster, such as a flood or fire.

It can be valuable to get a feel for major geographical moves undertaken in childhood. If someone was a "military brat," for example, and lived in many towns and cities, this can be of interest.

Family names are also important. We can often comment on the family traditions of names.

"I loved my father. His name was Tobe. I named our daughter, Toby, for him," Willa McCabe explained proudly.

Henrietta Frazier enjoys sharing the story about her name. "My father died before I was born, so my mother named me Henrietta, for my father. His name was Henry."

We can also comment on the many interesting names from the past: "Your father's name was Zachariah and your mother's name was America; isn't that interesting!" Although they are sometimes dreaded and disdained, nicknames are important to record. Also of note are affectionate names the *person* may have called his or her parents—mama, mother, ma, pa, daddy, or father.

We must learn the *person's* favorite activities, hobbies, and games from childhood. After all, most of us spent many hours as children playing. Sports certainly played a big role for many people, who might have played hockey, softball, or football. Playground games can be recalled and even reenacted. More serious recreational activities, such as playing a musical instrument or collecting stamps and coins, can also be part of a comprehensive life story.

Many of us retain vivid and pleasurable memories of childhood pets. Was there a special cat or dog in the *person's* childhood, perhaps a black cat named Midnight or a collie just like Lassie? A *person* may even have had a pet deer on an Idaho ranch. People who grew up in rural areas might recall memories of winning a ribbon for a prize animal at a state fair, or of a pig that the family loved too much to eat!

Adolescence

Adolescence is considered one of the most influential life stages. Key life events during this time can include graduating from junior and senior high, dating, getting the first car, and getting a first job. Adolescence is also a time when children gain greater independence from parents—the first steps to adulthood.

Education is often a good starting point when covering this part of a life story. It is always good to know what kind of educational experience the *person* had. Did he or she complete high school? In this age of advanced education, it is important to recall that, for many older adults, graduation from *junior* high school was a major event. Many of them might have been the first one in the family to obtain a high school diploma, often a source of great pride.

What other life events were associated with school? Many individuals might have had successful school experiences such as being on the football team or cheerleading squad, or winning the local spelling bee. Experiences such as high school proms are memorable, and often are photographed for scrapbooks, which can be retrieved and utilized as part of the life story.

Early modes of transportation evoke special memories. How did the *person* get to school—by bus, by car, or by foot, "walking miles in the snow"? What was the *person's* first car? One California day center director told the authors that a discussion of "my first car" was one of the center's most successful programs. Even participants with poor memory seemed to be able to recall the make and color of their first car and that car's first flat tire. One day center participant recalled his car's rumble seat, which drew blank stares from several younger members of the staff. "Does that have something to do with earthquakes?" one aide asked.

Jobs are often the most important way people define themselves.

Most older adults with dementia started working in tough times—the Great Depression and World War II—when hours were long and wages were low. A complete life story should discuss the *person's* first job. It can be interesting to ask what the *person's* first wage was. Many young people would certainly be surprised to hear that a wage of several dollars *a week* was not uncommon!

Perhaps a fitting way to end the written life story of this exuberant period is to ask the *person* if he or she can remember his or her first kiss. This question almost always evokes a laugh or a smile.

Young Adulthood

Education, work, and family life often dominate the young adult years. Of course we want to obtain information about whether the *person* married and if he or she has children or grandchildren. Information about the *person's* spouse and children can be added to the family tree begun earlier. If the *person* remained single, we might find out more about any siblings to which he or she remained close, and whether there were nieces or nephews or special cousins who made up the extended family of the *person*.

Many individuals seek higher education during this period or begin working. A good life story incorporates the *person's* higher education (if any) and describes early work or career choices.

A wedding can be a highlight of this time of life, and a life story should include information about the wedding ceremony, especially any funny stories that can be recounted, such as the groom misplacing the ring or a multilevel cake that collapsed. Wedding pictures, part of most family's archives, can be a marvelous source of family history.

We should obtain as much information as we can about the job or career of the *person*. Was the *person* a doctor, farmer, day laborer, homemaker, electrician, or artist? Any collections or materials from the *person's* work that might still be available can be noted. An architect might still have his or her drawings. A homemaker might have kept an elaborate card file of recipes. We can make note of whether the *person* wore special clothing associated with his or her occupation, such as a military uniform, chef's apron, farmer's overalls, or nun's habit.

Some products might have a corporate logo that is meaningful to the *person*. A *person* might very much enjoy wearing an old workplace cap or looking at letterhead with a company logo. Sometimes employee personnel manuals, military discharge papers, diplomas, licenses, or other documents can be found that are important artifacts of a *person's* career.

Often, this period is one in which the *person* purchased his or her first home, an act that has enormous symbolic value. When possible, pictures of the first house should be included in the life story. A surprising number of *persons* with dementia may still remember the amount of their first monthly mortgage payment. We can find out how many bedrooms the house had, what it looked like, and whether it had land surrounding it or was located on a small lot. Many people from rural backgrounds have vivid memories of the outhouse.

Middle Age

Writing a complete life story of a person's middle-age period could fill several books, but again we want to highlight major themes to better understand the past of the *person* with Alzheimer's disease. Middle age is a period in life when a *person* typically reaches the peak of his or her career. What was his or her last job before retirement, and was there any noteworthy achievement? It can be important to understand whether the *person's* identity is tied to his or her job. Some people identify themselves first and foremost as a doctor, engineer, plumber, or farmer. For others, job and work were secondary to their identity as father, wife, brother, or stepmother.

Avocations often develop during this time. We should find out what hobbies the individual had or what recreational activities he or she enjoyed. Golfers often have spent countless hours thinking, talking, and sometimes anguishing over their game. If the *person* was a golfer (or still golfs), did he or she ever hit a hole in one?

We should also find out what happened during this time to the *person's* family. Did children marry? Were there grandchildren? Were there family reunions?

During the 1920s–1940s, adult fraternities, sororities, or societies were more popular than they are in the 1990s. As part of the life story, we should determine whether the *person* joined the Elks, Kiwanis, Moose, Daughters of the Nile, or other groups.

Later Years

For many people, retirement provides a chance to pursue a hobby or activity more avidly; the individual who played bridge only once a month can now play three times a week. Another can go salmon fishing every other day during the season. For many people, gardening is a pleasurable activity, and the life story should note their favorite flowers and whether they had special success with vegetables. Perhaps one year there was an 80-pound pumpkin in the garden!

Did the *person* have an active retirement period? Former President Jimmy Carter's mother, Miss Lillian, joined the Peace Corps at age 70. What a mistake it would have been for a biographer to leave out this fact when describing her life!

Did the *person* remain physically active? Some older adults in the 1990s work out at health clubs, bike across the country, or take weekly organized hiking trips. If he or she decided to spend the retirement years sitting on the front porch watching the world go by, a note can be made to tease about the rocking chair that occupied his or her day.

Retirement is often a time for travel, and a special vacation can still be a vivid memory even in a *person* with dementia. Was there one "dream-of-a-lifetime" trip or a yearly vacation spot? What was the special attraction—a tropical island or a desert hideaway? Are pictures or souvenirs available that can be utilized for the life story?

Many retired people volunteer in their communities. Find out if the *person* volunteered in a hospital auxiliary, for a local nonprofit organization, or for a church or youth group. Noting someone's contributions to the community in a life story can be very valuable. For example, a day center might even take a field trip to tour the library building named after a participant.

Some retired people use this period to enrich their lives through continuing education—formal or informal. Find out if the *person* was a reader, learned any new skills during this time, or developed a new business.

Other Major Ingredients

Certainly an important part of any life story is the *person's* cultural, religious, and ethnic background and what role this background played in his or her life. Is the individual Jewish and did he or she keep kosher and attend synagogue or temple? Were there family traditions celebrating the *person's* African American heritage? Did the *person's* grandfather move to California when that state was still part of Mexico? Conversely, it is also important to note if someone has no strong religious background. Perhaps he or she would feel uncomfortable singing gospel songs at the facility.

One often-overlooked part of a life story is a *person's* awards or major achievements. Winning a prize or award is such a major event to individuals that it remains in the memory longer than many other events. Therefore, we should try to learn if the *person* was honored with a Silver Star during World War II, a Volunteer of the Year award, or a Teacher of the Year award.

It is valuable to ask the *person* or his or her family additional questions to try to get to know the *person* well. Did he or she have any strong likes or dislikes? At a day center group, the authors discovered that one participant had answered that question, "Republicans," and another in the same group replied, "Democrats." We tried to steer clear of politics that day.

Some people have their own special "trademark" phrases such as "You bet!" or "Two heads are better than one." It can add flavor to the *person's* life story to know the special phrases that he or she often used.

An important part of the life story is the kind of food the *person* enjoyed or enjoys. Many people spend a lot of time thinking about food. Some pride themselves on knowing special recipes or on knowing how to cook foods reflecting their ethnicity. Food can still be a source of much enjoyment and sensory pleasure for the *person*.

We also should know a *person's* favorite song or type of music. It is important to let people listen to music they enjoy, whether it be Bach, Benny Goodman, or the Beatles.

Although it seems unimportant, we should ask what the *person's* favorite color is. Often, late into dementia a *person* can still respond to questions about color and is pleased to be surrounded by items or wear clothing of a favored color.

Sometimes a *person* will seem to favor the company of one gender over another. Did the *person* have mostly female or male friends?

The life story should also include any of the *person's* special skills. For example, often a *person* will retain the ability to play a beautiful old song that he or she has played for many years, despite the fact that Alzheimer's disease prevents him or her from learning a simple new song. Other common skills include cooking, sewing, painting, and making crafts.

Sometimes harder to determine but also important is the overall personality of the individual before developing Alzheimer's disease.

Learning this information is important because old personality patterns often are retained. Was he or she generally optimistic or pessimistic? What was his or her problem-solving approach? How was stress handled?

The authors recommend that a *person's* life story be updated regularly. Have there been any major family developments, such as weddings, reunions, or new grandchildren? Has the *person* gone on a trip? Has the family given the *person* a new pet?

The life story should take special note of any successes or happy memories that can be used to benefit the *person*. It should also offer warnings against any painful subjects, phobias, or important information to be avoided, if possible.

The following special notes should be made about compiling the life story:

- Inevitably there will be gaps in the life story because family members may not be available to answer questions and the *person* may be an unreliable reporter. If this is the case, we must do the best we can. No matter how many holes or mysteries, we are sure to find some nuggets of gold while writing the story.

- Unconventional questions about the *person* can be asked to add extra richness to the life story. For example, a day center director writing a life story might ask the family if the *person* might have held on to the first dollar earned or spent it the minute it came in. "Questions that Enrich a Written Life Story" (p. 76) provides a short list of sample questions.

- If the *person* believes things about his or her life that are not factually correct, they should be written into the story anyway. The authors do not encourage emphasizing these inaccuracies, but if some of this information is real to the *person*, we should be prepared to accept the new information and incorporate it into our plan of care.

Once, in the day program, Judge Jean Auxier signed his name "Senator Jean Auxier." Staff members asked his wife if he had ever been a Kentucky state senator, thinking they had missed an important achievement in his written life story. The wife expressed surprise, and said, "No, but he had always wanted to be!" Staff usually called Jean by his formal title, "Judge," but occasionally slipped in "Senator." This pleased him very much. He won the "election" without ever campaigning!

Questions that Enrich a Written Life Story

The authors always recommend "playing detective" when writing a life story. Looking beneath the surface can pay many dividends in knowing the *person* with Alzheimer's disease better. Unusual questions can reveal much about the *person's* attitudes toward life. The questions can be asked of friends and family or directly of the *person,* when possible. Because we are hoping to get an idea of the *person's* values before the onset of Alzheimer's disease, the questions are written in the past tense, but whenever possible we should obtain present-day answers as well.

1. How would the *person* have enjoyed spending New Year's Eve? It can be revealing to know if he or she would have been in the middle of Times Square, out dancing, or home with a book.

2. Did the *person* have a favorite book? It would be interesting to know whether he or she preferred a good mystery novel, Shakespeare, the Bible, poetry, an auto repair manual, or the Farmer's Almanac.

3. If the *person* was stuck on a desert island, what three things would he or she wish to have with him or her? (Assume that there is food, drink, and shelter.)

4. How would the *person's* desk have been organized? (If the person did not have a desk, substitute kitchen shelves and drawers, tool box, or barn.)

5. Would the *person* have looked at life thinking the glass is half-full (optimist) or half-empty (pessimist)?

6. Would the *person* have held onto the first dollar he or she made, or would it have "burned a hole" in his or her pocket?

The Best Friends Approach to Alzheimer's Care, by Virginia Bell and David Troxel.
Copyright © 1997, by Health Professions Press, Inc., Baltimore.

How to Utilize the Life Story

All of the elements of the life story provide important tools for improving communication, making activities meaningful, preventing problems, and adding more enjoyment to a caregiver's relationship with the individual with dementia. Some of the primary ways to utilize the life story are discussed below.

Greeting the *Person* and Improving Recognition

Depending on the severity of the dementia, the *person* may or may not recognize even a familiar day center staff member, family member, or friend. Without recognition, the opening moments of any interaction can be difficult. The *person* may become alarmed if he or she feels threatened (Who is this woman approaching me? Does she want to hurt me or rob me?), embarrassed (I should know this woman, but . . .), or simply unresponsive.

When the *person's* life story has been mastered by a caregiver, establishing recognition becomes easy. Consider the following example. A day center bus driver arrives at the home of a client to pick her up in the morning. The driver knows that the woman can sometimes be nervous and reluctant to leave. He starts the interaction by smiling, extending a warm handshake or touch, and introducing himself: "Hi, Mary! I'm John, your bus driver from the senior center." If John knows Mary's life story, he can add something such as, "I see you are wearing that pretty pink dress. I remember that pink has always been your favorite color." Then he might add, "How is your grandson Ed? Is he still on the high school football team?"

At the day center, staff and volunteers often greet Ruby Lee Chiles with a question such as, "Ruby Lee, how is Delbert, that handsome son of yours? You must be so proud of him. He's a master electrician!"

Utilizing elements from the life story in opening greetings promotes better recognition. In these examples, facts from the life story put the *persons* immediately at ease.

Introducing the *Person* to Others

Pam Richards is a day center director whose father was a participant in her program. She often introduced him to others with great fanfare and flourish: "Hello, everyone! I'd like you to meet my father, Vern Clark. He's a great guy. I know you'll enjoy meeting him."

The *person* can also be introduced with a biographical fact such as, "I'd like you to meet my friend who was born in London." These kinds of introductions serve two primary purposes. First, they build self-esteem and evoke smiles, sometimes putting the *person* at ease in uncomfortable social situations. Second, the *person* is introduced to others as a valued member of society, someone good to know.

Debate continues about whether to address someone by a proper name, such as Mr. Johnson, or by a first name. Although the authors believe that the *person* with Alzheimer's disease is best addressed by a first name, the life story will give important information about this subject. If someone is from the South, where society is more formal than that in southern California, it is possible that he or she would prefer to be introduced in a more formal fashion, such as "Mr." or "Mrs." Jones, or like "Miss" Lillian, former President Carter's mother, who was from Georgia. Jean Auxier certainly was used to, and expected to be addressed as, "Judge."

Recognizing one's own name is often one of the last cognitive skills lost to Alzheimer's disease. The authors recommend using the *person's* name often, be it a proper name or a name defining a relationship ("dad" or "sis"). It gets attention, reinforces the relationship with the *person*, and sometimes comforts the *person*.

Making introductions in a group setting, such as an activities class in a long-term care facility or a day center is an art. During a group activity, staff can go around the circle or room and "reintroduce" everyone, each time adding some small piece of biographical information. For example, if the group is tossing a ball around a circle, when each *person* catches the ball, the director of the activity can say, "Okay, now the ball is for Dicy. Dicy has a granddaughter named Nawanta." These few words draw Dicy's attention to the activity and increase her interest in continuing to play the game. The fact that the day center director has something special to say about everyone as the activity progresses promotes individual self-esteem while building group cohesiveness.

Reminiscing

Perhaps the most obvious benefit to having a good, comprehensive biography of the *person* is to allow for reminiscence. The sharing of memories and old stories is something that all of us enjoy; we may be able to tell an old story with great detail, and of course, usually with a number of embellishments (think of the classic fish stories).

Persons with Alzheimer's disease still enjoy reminiscing. When looking at an old family photograph, the person may, with cueing, be able to recall some names and relationships. If not, the photograph can still be used to talk about fashions from that era ("Mom, look at the hats ladies used to wear!") or to discuss other interesting items in the photograph ("Mom, is that lady really wearing a foxtail fur piece?").

Memories and impressions of parents and grandparents often remain vivid.

Mary Burmaster loves to be reminded that her grandfather was a beloved country doctor. Staff members at her day center remind her about her grandfather and then they reminisce together, not so much about the details of her grandfather's life but about country doctors in general. They talk about doctors delivering babies, their black bags, and that they wish physicians still made house calls. Whenever possible, staff incorporate details they know about her grandfather. "Mary, I remember you telling me that his first house call was way back at the turn of the century!"

Early childhood stories, particularly ones involving childhood mischievousness, are enjoyable to the person. Gently teasing a retired college professor about how he used to skip school can bring laughter. A day center participant can be reminded of the time he took his uncle's wool hat and stuck it up the chimney to hide it, only to be found out when a fire was lit and the room filled with smoke!

Margaret Brubaker enjoyed being reminded (and teased) about the times she would play the game of craps. She even taught her son Jim how to play. Because she always greeted visitors in such a proper manner and appeared to be very traditional, it was fun to reminisce with her about this hidden and unexpected talent.

Improving Communication through Clues and Cues

The impact of dementia on language skills can be severe. Often, individuals with Alzheimer's disease use incorrect words, lose words, and in general have trouble communicating. Knowing the life story can improve communication because the life story may provide clues to aid in understanding what the person is saying. For example, if someone with dementia says, "I need to get home, the children, it's getting late," a caregiver who is familiar with the *person's* life story might recall that the *person* was a homemaker who made a big dinner for her family every night. The caregiver might make a guess and say, "Oh, Carol, don't worry. Your daughter Stephanie has already made a delicious dinner for everyone. Tonight *you* get to be spoiled."

The life story also helps us to provide clues, when needed, to allow the *person* to finish a sentence. If someone says, "I need to call my husband . . ." and is struggling to find his name, a caregiver can supply the name by saying, "You mean your husband, *Mike?*" If someone keeps talking about his or her childhood but seems unable to supply many details, you can utilize the life story to inquire, "Mary, it must have been wonderful growing up in the pretty town of Walla Walla. Aren't you lucky to have grown up surrounded by those beautiful wheat fields and famous sweet onions?"

Evelyn Talbott had an intense desire to converse. She lit up whenever someone would prompt her about her work, her love of dogs, her interest in dancing, and her enjoyable nature walks. She would use her hands to gesture toward her body, saying with her hands, "give me more, keep going." People who knew elements of her life story found it easy to converse with her, but someone who did not know much about her would find the conversation ended quickly. Evelyn needed others to do most of the work, to "carry the ball" in conversations.

Designing Appropriate Activities

The life story provides many important clues to activities that may have the greatest chance of capturing the *person's* interest and evoking a positive, joyful response. We can look to the *person's* life story for clues about his or her *skills*. For example, an accountant diagnosed with Alzheimer's disease certainly will no longer be able to handle a complex transaction, but he or she might enjoy "helping" to add a row of figures. One could ask a retired librarian to help organize a collection of magazine clippings and photographs. A former homemaker may enjoy helping to prepare a batch of cookies or folding laundry. A retired shoe salesperson may enjoy looking at wholesale shoe catalogs and "placing" a new order. The possibilities are endless.

Walter Turner always loved to play horseshoes. Staff at the adult day center made certain that he could still play an indoor version of the game whenever he wanted. It gave him great pleasure to give lessons to the other participants and staff. When he made a ringer, he always enjoyed the round of applause that followed.

Larkin Myers enjoyed teaching others how to "spin a top." He had retained his childhood skill of winding the string on the wooden top and then spinning it so it would whirl around for a seemingly impossible length of time.

Ruby Lee Chiles was raised with a very strong work ethic. She resists all activities that seem unproductive. Her life story allowed the staff of the adult day center she attends to shape a series of "jobs" for her. Even when she participates in a recreational activity such as an art project, staff members say, "Come on, Ruby Lee, there's work to do." Putting a crafts project into this context and asking her to "fix this," "fold this," and "straighten this" seems to motivate her to become more involved in the activity.

The life story provides a rich source of ideas for "show and tell." If the *person* had created crafts, collected stamps, painted, won bowling trophies, and so forth, the life story can note these items, which can then be used one-on-one to reminisce. Simply bringing in a collection of old neckties would probably fill an afternoon with discussion and laughter about the varying styles, colors, and widths that came into, out of, and back into fashion.

We should not forget that the most important of all activities is simply being with others. Many *persons* with dementia are starved for attention. Knowing the *person's* life story makes it possible for a volunteer, a professional, or even a family friend to better relate to and be with the *person*.

Pointing Out Past Accomplishments

We honor individuals with dementia by remembering their accomplishments.

Mary Katherine Davis still remembers that she did not like milking cows and getting up early on the farm. She was determined to get off the farm and went to school to become a nurse. This was always a source of great pride when mentioned in conversation.

The life story gives us information to be able to point out the accomplishments of family members; for example, almost all parents like hearing good things about their children. We can point out when someone's grandson is the star football player or congratulate the *person* if his or her daughter has just received a big promotion.

During the 1940s and 1950s, Marcus Powell had a reputation for growing some of the best garden produce in Iowa City, produce he would share freely with his colleagues and students. Years later he still enjoyed being reminded about his accomplished green thumb.

Helping to Prevent Challenging Behaviors

Many challenging behaviors are caused by identifiable triggers, such as being exposed to grandchildren who are too loud, being asked inappropriate questions, or being rushed. However, sometimes behaviors are hard to explain, and may stem from more deep-rooted concerns that might only be apparent from the *person's* life story.

Sometimes a behavior can be triggered when sad memories are inadvertently raised. For example, if a *person* lost family members in a boating accident, problems may occur if a volunteer in a day center shows photographs of his or her new boat. The *person* may not be able to explain his or her feelings, but instead might act out or become despondent. In that case, without a good life story, it is almost impossible to determine why the nautical discussions are making someone unhappy.

Brevard Crihfield was used to being the boss at work. He enjoyed the sing-along sessions at the day center until one week, when he became angry during the session. The song leader that day had a wonderful voice and was charismatic as he stood in front of the group. The group loved him. However, he was also somewhat directive, and "Crihf" read that as someone standing in front of him, telling him what to do. When the song leader sat by the piano to lead the songs instead of standing, Crihf's outbursts stopped.

A simple intervention led to a big payoff, because Crihf was calmed and the program could go on.

Geri Greenway found popular music distasteful. She enjoyed fine classical music and opera but could not abide the popular, nostalgic songs often sung in the day program. Staff quickly learned to distract Geri and let her do other things during the music hour.

Staff at Helping Hand were surprised one day when the usually affable Patsy Peck got angry and called the center director a "goody two-shoes." Later, staff members discussed what might have caused this outburst and turned to Patsy's life story for some clues. They realized that, as Director of Physical Therapy for a local hospital, Patsy had always been the "Good Samaritan," the person who helped others. Perhaps her outburst was related to her frustration at no longer being in this role. The staff began to ask Patsy to work with a new student in the program. The two quickly became inseparable, and Patsy was again enjoying the helping role.

Incorporating Past Daily Rituals

Some individuals have rituals in their daily life, whether it is going to Mass each morning, taking a daily walk, or, as the authors once read about a famous film director, having a chocolate malt every day at 2 P.M.! Daily rituals can be utilized in Alzheimer's disease care.

If a *person* enjoyed a daily newspaper and cup of coffee, let him or her start the day that way. Even when the *person* may not be able to fully read a paper or retain the content, there is enormous symbolic value in simply holding it and turning the pages. Reading a newspaper suggests to others that one is educated, informed, and interested in the world. Offering the *person* a cup of coffee is a social interaction as well as a gift, and the coffee's warmth and aroma may stimulate positive memories. One family told us that, when they discovered this ritual, it kept their father busy and satisfied for over an hour every morning.

Nancy Zechman loved nothing better than a long daily drive in the country. Often, Nancy climbed into her husband, Fred's, blue truck well before the scheduled time of 4 P.M., saying, "Let's go, Fred." This routine was especially effective with Nancy. Driving into the country was an activity that both Nancy and Fred enjoyed; it also relieved the anxiety that arises at a time of day that is stressful for many caregivers.

Beverly Wheeler has always enjoyed walking. She and her husband find that walking on the wood piers along California's central coast provides great exercise and a chance to smell the salty air, listen to the crashing waves, look for dolphins, and observe sea lions and pelicans. They have set a goal for themselves to walk every pier along the southern California coast—eventually maybe even the entire state.

Broadening the Caregiving Network and Resources

A life story can remind families, agencies, adult day center directors, and residential care facility operators of the richness of the *person's* past. In many cases the *person* volunteered in church groups or civic and social clubs. In some cases a *person* belonged to a special military unit, the police or fire department, or a trade union.

From the life story, a list can be made of potential organizations or volunteers who can provide help to the family or volunteer support to the service program. The local fire department can be asked to bring their mascot dalmatian to the nursing facility to visit a retired firefighter with dementia. A church organist can be asked to play for a member who can no longer attend services. A local service club can be asked to raise funds for a new adult day center that would benefit several of their members.

Because the day center staff knew that Nancy Zechman was an avid tennis player, they looked to her social contacts and friends for potential volunteer help. Her tennis partners at the Lexington Tennis Club were contacted, and Nancy's close friend, Jody Bollum, agreed to be with Nancy at the day center once a week. When together, Jody helped Nancy feel safe and secure, in part because they had many stories and experiences in common.

The next section presents the extended, written life story of Rebecca Matheny Riley, with comments on how it can be used to provide good care. The authors hope you will be pleased to get to know our friend Rebecca even better.

LIFE STORY OF REBECCA MATHENY RILEY

Rebecca is the oldest child [*talk about responsibility of firstborn*], born January 8, 1925, to Elsie Arnold and S.F. Matheny. She also has the distinction of being the first granddaughter on both sides of her family [*unique family story*]. Rebecca and her only sister, Mary Frances, 18 months younger, were very close as children and remain intimate friends [*likes talking about childhood stories*]. When Rebecca was only 3 years old, her mother died [*source of sadness*] and her grandparents became parents to Rebecca and her little sister.

Rebecca adored her grandparents and named them Grandpa and Grandma [*talk about names used to describe grandparents*]. Her grandmother came to this country in 1892 from Austria, and some family members still reside there.

The little girls were happy-go-lucky as they played in the creek that ran through their grandparents' farm. Catching frogs and tadpoles that lived in the creek was a favorite pastime on a hot summer day. On autumn days, they enjoyed gathering hickory nuts and walnuts [*reminisce about gathering nuts, talk about the tastes and uses of nuts*] that had fallen from the many trees on the farm.

Grandpa had lots of animals, including one horse that he allowed the little girls to ride alone. This horse was very slow and deliberate and always dependable as he carried the girls safely on his back. One day this trusty horse became frightened and, as he ran faster and faster, the girls held on "for dear life." Rebecca remembers the scary ride and how happy they were when a neighbor rescued them [*memorable story that made a big impact, can be repeated*].

Rebecca had many friends at school [*create a collage of school-related pictures*]. A favorite game to play with her classmates was the game of hide-and-seek [*Rebecca enjoys games—perhaps try charades*]. When Rebecca was in the first grade, she invited her entire class to come home with her after school [*tease her about this*]. This was a big surprise to Grandpa and Grandma. Although they all had a great time playing at the farm, she remembers a serious discussion about asking permission before inviting so many friends to visit [*discussion about discipline then and now*].

Rebecca and Mary Frances were often responsible for doing the dishes after supper to help their grandmother. They argued about whose turn it was to clean up the kitchen [*reminisce about chores*].

As Rebecca grew older, she wondered about her mother: "What was she really like?" "Why did she have to leave me when I was such a little girl?" Her father remarried and she now had two brothers, Sam and Earl. Although Grandma and Grandpa were wonderful "parents," Rebecca often had sad thoughts about not knowing her mother [*remember this if she expresses feelings of sadness; could be old feelings/ memories*].

Even as a young girl Rebecca was goal oriented. She had a determined spirit and a mind of her own, refusing to take "no" for an answer [*make note of this, speak in positives instead of in negatives*]. That spirit remains very much a part of her. She always wanted to be helpful, especially to others in great need. She was motivated to learn, making her an excellent student [*some key personality traits—motivated, goal oriented, helpful*]. During her youth, Rebecca was a member of the Methodist church and active in the Epworth League sponsored by the church. Her religious faith fed her spirit and desire to be helpful. She often made known her life goals: to be a nurse, serve as a missionary, and marry a minister [*religion is very important to her*].

During her years at Stanford High School, Rebecca played in the

The life story can be sup-
plemented with photo-
graphs of the *person.* At
left, Rebecca is pictured
from her childhood (seen
here with her younger
sister, Mary Frances)
through her early nursing
career, her marriage to Jo,
and her young adult-
hood, raising a family.

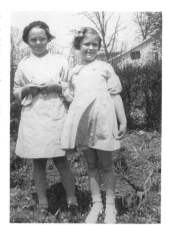

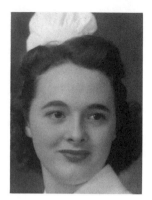

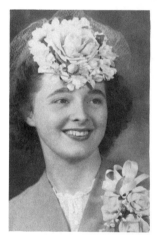

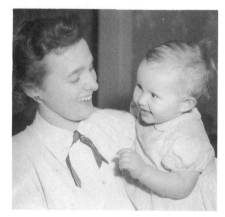

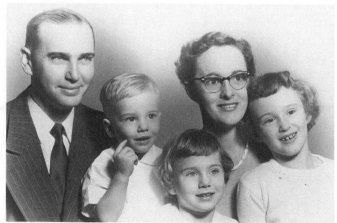

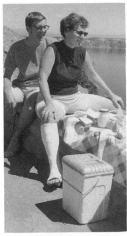
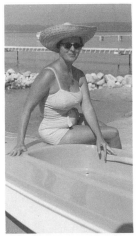
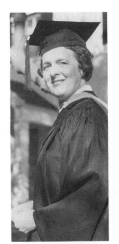
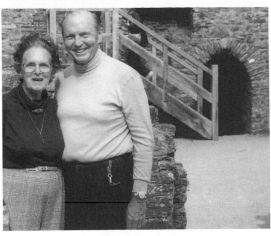
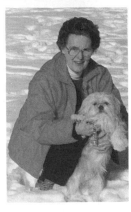
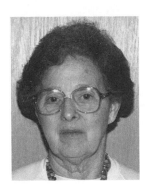

Rebecca enjoys the Grand Canyon even with a broken leg. She is pictured here relaxing by Crystal Lake, Michigan, and graduating with a bachelor's of science in nursing. As the dementia progressed, Rebecca found comfort in playing with Corky and traveling the world with Jo. According to Jo, she is totally dependent on continuous care at the Christian Health Care Center in Lexington, but as a close friend noted, "She still has those soft eyes and warm smile."

band [*check to see if she still plays any instruments*]. She was also a member of the Girl's Reserve Club and graduated with honors [*opportunity for congratulations*]. After graduation, she enrolled in nurse's training at Good Samaritan Hospital in Lexington, Kentucky. As a nursing student [*likes to be reminded she is a nurse, complimented on past achievements as a nurse*], she met her husband while he was a patient in the hospital [*funny story about how they met*]. Although nursing students at that time were not allowed to remain in school after marriage, Rebecca relied on her determined spirit [*determination*] and became the first married nursing student at the hospital [*note as major accomplishment*].

On April 20, 1945 she married Jo M. Riley, an ordained minister in the Christian church (Disciples of Christ) [*talk about wedding traditions*]. His pastorates took them to Kokomo, Indiana; Wilson, North Carolina; Decatur, Illinois; Louisville, Kentucky; and Centralia, Illinois. She taught church classes for children and young adults and was very supportive of all church activities. She served on a national Week of Compassion committee for her church [*compliment her on leadership ability*]. This was a special honor for Rebecca, giving her the opportunity to use her expertise on a national level [*this was a happy time for her*].

Rebecca was nominated Mother of the Year while living in Kokomo, Indiana, and was President of the Minister's Wives Organization of Illinois. These honors are very special to her. The community also benefited from Rebecca's helping hands. She was a Girl Scout leader for several years [*praise her for her contributions to the community*].

Rebecca and Jo became parents of three children, Lucinda, Joetta, and Louis [*use the names for conversational cues*]. Lucinda and her son Josh live in Washington, D.C. Joetta is married to William Parris and lives in North Carolina. Louis and his wife, Joy, have three children, Ian, Tristan, and Grant. They live in Tennessee. Rebecca has always been family oriented; her family comes first [*any mention of her family always makes her feel special and proud*].

Rebecca and Jo own a cottage on Crystal Lake in Michigan. Each summer the family vacationed there [*could be the source of old photos or mementos, fun memories*]. Given an hour's notice, Rebecca said they could be packed up and ready to go. This was a wonderful place for the children to play [*talk about her children's experiences each summer at the lake*]. The cottage was located just a stone's throw from the water. Swimming and enjoying their rowboat were great ways for the family to spend time together. Also, family and friends returned each year to nearby cottages. Often, these friends gathered with the Riley family for picnics at special locations on the lake. One of Rebecca's favorite activities was a breakfast picnic on a hot summer day. The sand dunes nearby were very tall and inviting to climb after the picnic [*tease her that she exercised so hard after a big meal*].

Cooking is an art to Rebecca. Wherever she lived, she learned how to prepare local dishes and delighted in serving these dishes to visitors to the community. Two Rebecca specialties were "popcorn" cake and persimmon pudding [*she may enjoy being asked her opinion about recipes, tasting unusual dishes*]. Rebecca remembers preparing a reception for 500 people—what a big task!

In 1972 Rebecca returned to school to earn a bachelor's of science degree in nursing, and in 1974 she received a master's degree in education from Spaulding College. She taught nursing students until she was diagnosed with Alzheimer's disease in July 1984. Spaulding College, Jefferson Community College, and Centralia College all benefited from her gift of teaching [*likes to do things that evoke skills of teaching*].

After their children were grown, Jo and Rebecca traveled to England, Scotland, Australia, New Zealand, Israel and Jordan, China, Russia, Austria, and other European countries. While in Austria, they visited Rebecca's grandmother's home, the fulfillment of a dream for Rebecca [*pictures, mementos?*].

Rebecca also enjoys classical music, knitting, sewing, reading, and homemaking. Her favorite hymn is "Amazing Grace." Her dog, Corky, is a constant companion, especially since the diagnosis of Alzheimer's disease. Corky reminds her of her childhood pet dog, Briar [*all good activity ideas*].

The following update, dated April 1996, was given to the authors by Rebecca's family.

When Rebecca was diagnosed she wanted to be told of her diagnosis. She shared her feelings about the result openly and honestly as long as she was able to do so. Rebecca wanted to do everything she could to be of help to others. She was particularly interested in doing her part to further research into the cause(s) of Alzheimer's disease. Rebecca is currently a resident of the Christian Health Care Center in Lexington, Kentucky. Her husband was her primary caregiver at home for many years and continues to visit her daily to be with her and provide supplemental care. Rebecca is totally dependent but, as a close friend noted, "She still has those soft eyes and warm smile."

CONCLUSION

The life story is a key element of the Best Friends model of care. Good Alzheimer's care must be *individualized* care. The life story helps us create a special, caring, one-on-one relationship with everyone we deal with who has Alzheimer's disease, whether he or she is at home, in a day center, or even in a large nursing facility.

Creating a life story has another important value: For the *person* and the family, the life story is a way of recording one's life achievements. When families come together to create the document, the life story can be a healing tool. It can be a celebration of someone's life. It can be a document to tuck into the family Bible for generations to come.

Medical science has developed prostheses for people who have lost limbs, techniques to bring back eyesight for people with cataracts, and devices to improve hearing. Although there is no cure or treatment for *people* with Alzheimer's disease, we do have a method of bringing back memories—*a human prosthesis*, Best Friends. Best Friends are their memory, their biographer.

7

The "Knack" of Alzheimer's Care

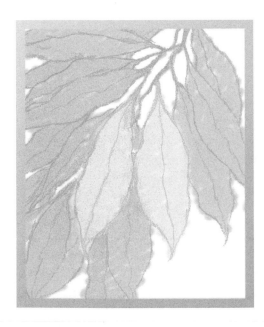

In support groups and at conferences throughout the United States, there is a new sense of optimism about progress in medical and scientific research in Alzheimer's disease. Yet family and professional caregivers still search for help to learn how to provide care, still face daily failures, and still cope with the challenges of providing high-quality institutional care. At the authors' U.S. speaking engagements, the common concerns we have heard include the following:

I stayed up 2 hours past my normal bedtime planning a 3-hour craft activity for my mother and the whole project was over in 5 minutes.

I feel like I've run out of ideas to do at the day center. My program is getting stale.

The nursing home aides work so hard, but they just don't seem to be able to connect with my husband.

At the same time we hear about these problems and concerns, it seems that wherever we travel we meet people, such as the following, who seem to have a "magic touch" in their work with, or care of, people with Alzheimer's disease:

- The beloved nursing assistant who can rise to any occasion and always seems to say or do the right thing.
- The husband who gives loving care to his wife, uses local services, and approaches his tasks in a joyful way, seemingly avoiding the burnout that affects so many caregivers.
- The day center activities director who is always coming up with ideas for a consistently rich and innovative activity program.

What is the difference between these two types of caregivers? Some caregivers have more financial resources to draw on, which can make a positive difference. A large and supportive family can help. In professional settings the budget and number of volunteers can enrich programs. Yet some caregivers and some institutions with almost-unlimited resources still fail to provide good care, while others with no resources thrive.

The difference is that the latter type of care provider has mastered the *knack* of caregiving. The word "knack" is defined as a clever trick or stratagem or the ability and skill to do something easily. Some individuals are simply born with knack; their personality and sensibility help them to be wonderful caregivers. The Best Friends model can teach the abilities and skills of knack and along the way offer many clever tricks in the "dos and don'ts" of Alzheimer's care.

ELEMENTS OF KNACK

The knack of caring for a *person* with Alzheimer's disease is composed of many skills and abilities (also listed on the form "Elements of Knack," p. 94). This section discusses the elements of knack that are central to the Best Friends model of care.

Being Well-Informed

Caregivers with knack learn as much as they can about Alzheimer's disease in order to be better informed of new research and treatments, to learn caregiving tips, and to locate new community resources. They attend conferences and workshops, subscribe to appropriate newsletters, and talk to other families coping with dementia. They know that the more one knows about Alzheimer's disease the less stressful the difficult job of caregiving becomes.

Having Empathy

Caregivers with knack have taken time to imagine what it would be like to have Alzheimer's disease. This helps them understand the world of the *person* they care about or care for and how that world can be difficult and frightening. Empathy also teaches that the *person's* world is very real to him or her, and that problems that come up may be caused by the *person's* attempts to cope logically with his or her world.

Respecting the Basic Rights of the *Person*

Caregivers with knack regard people with Alzheimer's disease as human beings with infinite value, people who deserve loving, high-quality care. They embrace the Alzheimer's Disease Bill of Rights not as a formal, legal document but rather as a statement of goals. They give the *person* as much say in his or her care as possible and try to keep him or her productive in work and play as long as possible.

Maintaining Caregiving Integrity

Caregivers with knack approach problems and decision making with an attitude of good will toward the *person,* and they approach care in an ethical fashion. When they withhold information or work their way out of problematic situations, they do so out of concern and in the best interests of the *person.* For example, a caregiver who decides not to tell her mother that they are going to visit an adult day center for the first time and "surprises" her mother with the visit may in fact be withholding information, but this decision is made with caregiving integrity.

Employing Finesse

Caregivers with knack are able to utilize the art of finesse to respond to difficult situations. They use skillful, subtle, tactful, diplomatic, and well-timed maneuvers to handle problems. In the game of bridge a finesse is taking a trick economically. The same holds true in Alzheimer's care; as caregivers we want to win a few hands. Thus, if a *person* says, "I want to go home," and we respond, "Soon," we are using finesse to give the *person* the answer he or she wants to hear.

ELEMENTS OF KNACK

Being well-informed

Having empathy

Respecting the basic rights of the *person*

Maintaining caregiving integrity

Employing finesse

Knowing it is easier to get forgiveness
    than to get permission

Using common sense

Communicating skillfully

Maintaining optimism

Setting realistic expectations

Using humor

Employing spontaneity

Maintaining patience

Developing flexibility

Staying focused

Being nonjudgmental

Valuing the moment

Maintaining self-confidence

Using cueing tied to the life story

Taking care of oneself

Planning ahead

The Best Friends Approach to Alzheimer's Care, by Virginia Bell and David Troxel.
Copyright © 1997, by Health Professions Press, Inc., Baltimore.

We hope the *person* will move on to another subject. If someone wants to know where his wife is and she is deceased, a change of subject done with finesse can prove helpful. Some family members struggle with this strategy, feeling that they are lying or being deceitful. As long as caregiver integrity is maintained, the authors believe that skillful finesse is part of good Alzheimer's care.

Knowing it Is Easier to Get Forgiveness than to Get Permission

Caregivers with knack know that sometimes decisions must be made for the *person*. Caregivers at times must be decisive. They know that asking permission works with a person whose cognitive abilities are unimpaired but is not always the best idea when someone has dementia. Thus, when the *person* needs an appointment with his or her doctor, it is often best for the caregiver to make the arrangements and withstand some temporary upset if he or she achieves the goal. Usually, the *person* will forget about the incident, in effect forgiving the caregiver for making the appointment without permission. When the *person* does become angry or upset at the caregiver for making this decision, the caregiver may find it expedient to simply "take the blame" to maintain peace and to "save face" for the person.

Using Common Sense

Caregivers with knack exercise common sense. They are not afraid to seek simple solutions to complex problems. Examples of common sense ideas the authors have heard from caregivers include eliminating caffeine when the *person* has problems sleeping, making extra sets of keys in case a set is hidden or lost, having the *person* wear an identification bracelet, and making extra photographs of the *person* in case of wandering.

Communicating Skillfully

Caregivers with knack communicate skillfully, cueing the *person* with appropriate words from his or her life story, using positive body language, and knowing the right and wrong ways to ask and answer questions. Good communication also involves skilled listening, and the best caregivers work hard to help the *person* better communicate. More ideas for communication are discussed in Chapter 8.

Maintaining Optimism

Caregivers with knack try to look beyond Alzheimer's disease and remember the good things in life. They take joy in even small pleasures that can come from time spent with their loved one with dementia. Caregivers maintain a sense of hope that the future will be brighter and that one day a cure for Alzheimer's disease will be found. They try to instill this sense of optimism and hope in the *person* with the disease.

Setting Realistic Expectations

Caregivers with knack have given thought to what the *person* can still do. Utilizing the assessment form discussed in Chapter 3 the caregiver can determine the *person's* remaining cognitive strengths, the state of his or her physical health, and other factors that affect everyday life and care. Expectations that are too high or too low can be frustrating to both caregiver and *person*.

Using Humor

Caregivers with knack are not afraid to tell funny stories and jokes, or laugh when humorous things happen. They understand that even when the *person* does not "get" a funny story or joke, laughter and good feelings are contagious. The *person* will absorb these good feelings. Another key element of humor is that caregivers should not be afraid to make fun of themselves. Self-deprecation preserves dignity and is a small price to pay to make the *person* feel better about his or her own circumstances.

Employing Spontaneity

Caregivers with knack are not afraid to be spontaneous. A day planned for planting vegetables might also include an hour of unplanned bird-watching when colorful cardinals are spotted in the trees. People with Alzheimer's disease live in a world full of spontaneous events. If the *person* becomes interested in the color of a car or a particular object in the house, go with the flow!

Maintaining Patience

Caregivers with knack realize that it takes the *person* longer to do things and longer to respond to words and events. The act of dressing can take an hour, but it may be an hour during which the *person* is focused and does not feel lost and/or lonely. If the caregiver does not have an hour to spend dressing the *person,* creative solutions can make life run smoother (e.g., using clothes with Velcro fasteners or simplified outfits). All caregivers occasionally lose their patience, but getting frustrated and angry tends to make matters worse.

Developing Flexibility

Caregivers with knack recognize that the best-planned schedule cannot be set in stone because the *person* may in fact have his or her own ideas about how the day will transpire. It is important to examine oneself and develop greater flexibility as a caregiver. Some individuals have lived their lives with great discipline, getting things done on time and adhering to a schedule. This can be a recipe for disaster as a caregiver. Standards may have to be changed, but never need to be lowered.

Staying Focused

Caregivers with knack learn the importance of focus. With all the distractions around us, it can be hard at times to give the *person* the attention needed to provide good care. This is particularly challenging in long-term care and day center settings, where many things are happening at once. A nursing assistant, for example, should always focus on the activity of giving someone a bath, not on talking about how a friend did not show up for a date. The knack of focus involves really listening to and seeing the *person,* and getting the most out of every interaction. It also involves putting the caregiver's own concerns or problems on hold during this time. Anxiety, for example, can show up in facial expression or in vocal tones and can be misread or misunderstood by the *person.*

Being Nonjudgmental

Caregivers with knack work on being nonjudgmental toward the *person,* family and friends, and themselves. Stress and strain is inherent in caregiving, and friends and family may not always be present when needed, may say the wrong thing, or may let the caregiver down. Of course, it can be very easy to be angry at or disappointed in the *person* despite the caregiver's best intentions. Caregivers may not always be at their best and must learn not to be too hard on themselves.

Valuing the Moment

Caregivers with knack know the importance of living in and valuing the moment. A pleasant lunch, time spent arranging flowers, or a joyful game may soon be forgotten, but it can be pleasurable for everyone in the moment. If caregivers can learn to string together these positive moments, good Alzheimer's care can be achieved.

Maintaining Self-Confidence

Caregivers with knack exhibit self-confidence in their interactions with the *person*. The authors hope that the Best Friends model will, in fact, help instill this confidence. To be confident, we need to feel that we know what we are doing, have a plan of action, and have some successes to make us feel that we are doing the right thing. Often, this inner strength can be sensed by the *person,* who may then let go of his or her own concerns or fears. Conversely, if caregivers, family members, or professionals are tentative in their actions, the *person* may sense these feelings and become uneasy.

Using Cueing Tied to the Life Story

Caregivers with knack are able to incorporate the life story into all aspects of care, cueing the *person* to remember certain names, places, and things; telling familiar stories; and reminding him or her of past achievements.

Taking Care of Oneself

Caregivers with knack do not wait too long to use important local services such as adult day centers, home help, and home-delivered meals. All caregivers with knack try to find time for themselves, to maintain friendships, exercise, eat well, and not let their identity become wrapped up in the caregiving role. More information about being one's own best friend is provided in Chapter 13.

Planning Ahead

Caregivers with knack plan ahead for activities and utilize services, meals, and other aspects of care. Also, caregivers with knack have made it a priority to put the *person's* financial and legal affairs in order. This process should include a contingency plan in case the caregiver becomes incapacitated or dies. Who will then care for the *person*?

These are important decisions that should not be neglected by the primary caregiver.

THE BEST FRIENDS MODEL

This section reviews the Best Friends model as described in the book thus far. Remember that the Best Friends model will help us to develop the knack of good care.

It is revealing to look at some traditional dictionary definitions of the word "model" and see how the Best Friends model fits in. Table 3 delineates the fit. The Best Friends model is like a set of plans, an analogy, a pattern, or an example to help build caregiving skills. The Best Friends model is a road map to get professional and family caregivers from "here" to "there." The model offers many different routes to the destination. The result is that the caregiver with knack will be a "model caregiver," one who is able to help bring out the best in the *person* he or she cares about, one who can provide care with self-confidence and has the ability to make the best of almost any situation. The authors review the destinations along this road map in Table 4.

Prerequisites

Knowing the Basics

Although caregivers do not need to have extensive medical or scientific knowledge about Alzheimer's disease, the authors encourage them to learn as much as they can. For the purposes of the Best Friends model, it is particularly important to obtain a thorough workup to understand that the disease's impact on cognition is real, and to learn the concept of "excess disability."

Assessing Strengths and Having Appropriate Expectations

The goal of an assessment is to tell us who the *person* is and of what he or she is still capable. Family members and professional caregivers who set expectations too high are bound to find themselves frustrated and disappointed. Those who set expectations too low will see an increase in problems because the *person* might become bored with or angry or agitated about his or her lack of involvement in day-to-day activities. It is important to also remember that, under the Best Friends model, we do not want to allow an assessment to label someone too

Table 3.   Definition of "model"

Standard definitions	Best Friends model
A set of plans for a building	A plan for building caregiving skills
An analogy to help visualize something	An analogy to help caregivers visualize another approach
A pattern to be followed	A pattern for repeated successes
An example for imitation or emulation	An example to help the caregiver to develop knack, to be a person whom others emulate

narrowly because labeling might stifle spontaneity or creative care approaches.

Valuing Basic Rights

The authors encourage caregivers to embrace the Alzheimer's Disease Bill of Rights for dementia care. Families should utilize this list of rights (see p. 38) as a starting point for discussions about care, incorporating the list's philosophy into everyday care. Administrators of institutions should incorporate the Alzheimer's Disease Bill of Rights into their programs and care plans, not as another set of regulations but rather as a statement of goals. Ultimately, the value of the Alzheimer's Disease Bill of Rights is to remind us of the value of the *person* we care for—certainly an essential ingredient of knack.

Considering the Ingredients of Good Friendships

Elements of good friendship can teach us much about Alzheimer's care. Such elements include knowing each other's background and traditions, understanding individual personality, doing things together, initiating activities, providing encouragement, building self-esteem, listening well, giving compliments, asking opinions, enjoying old stories, laughing together, having a sense of equality, living with the ups and downs, and, above all, working at the relationship.

Knowing the *Person's* Life Story Well

A comprehensive knowledge of the *person's* life story can serve us well for all aspects of dementia care. Because *persons* with Alzheimer's disease cannot tell their life stories, we must become their biographers. Knowing a life story is much more complex than learning simple facts

Table 4.   The Best Friends model of Alzheimer's care: A road map to success

Prerequisites	Applying change	Result
Knowing the basics (see Chapter 2)		
Assessing strengths and having appropriate expectations (see Chapter 3)		
Valuing basic rights (see Chapter 4)	Recasting relationships →	KNACK
Considering the ingredients of good friendships (see Chapter 5)		
Knowing the *person's* life story well (see Chapter 6)		

and dates. We want to know about the person's values, past goals and dreams, and special accomplishments. Of note is that the life story is ongoing; current events should be incorporated so that they can be woven into daily activities or care whenever appropriate.

Applying Change: Recasting Relationships

Family caregivers coping with Alzheimer's disease are often dismayed at the change in their relationships with the *person*. Rather than staying in a state of despair, they can recast their relationships with the *person* to embrace a model of friendship—they can become Best Friends. Professionals should also recast their relationships and work to treat their resident or day center participant as though they were good friends.

Professionals may face a different challenge in recasting relationships. Adult day center and long-term care facility administrators may need to look at job descriptions, scheduling, staff training, and statements of philosophy or mission statements to try to effect organizational change. One challenge is to become people oriented instead of task oriented.

Result: The Knack

Caregivers who successfully learn the Best Friends model of care will develop knack, or the *ability to do something easily,* and will learn many tricks along the way. Knack for families is all about resilience, about surviving the disease, about providing good care, and about enjoying moments with the *person*. It is about the quality of life, for the *person* and his or her loved ones. It is about working through the pain. One door is closing and another is opening.

KNACK IN ALZHEIMER'S CARE

This section outlines some common scenarios caregivers encounter when dealing with individuals with Alzheimer's disease. A number of situations are presented comparing Alzheimer's care with "no knack" and with "knack." These examples show readers how the Best Friends model can be applied to typical situations. Some of the common threads running through all the examples are good listening, empathy, humor, creativity, skilled communication, and lots of patience. As noted earlier, if we have met one *person* with Alzheimer's disease, we have met only one *person* with Alzheimer's disease; every case is somewhat different. Thus, the following examples may or may not be appropriate to a given situation. The authors hope that readers will be inspired by these examples of knack, or Alzheimer's care at its best, and apply the lessons to their own situations.

★ Coping with Forgetting

A common complaint to a family member might be "I just cannot remember anything! What are my grandchildren's names?"

No-Knack Approach

"You'll be better soon. Don't worry about it."

Example of Knack

"It must be difficult to forget the things you most want to remember. Let me write down the names of your grandchildren for you."

Discussion

Many people with Alzheimer's disease recognize their memory losses and express frustration at times with not being able to retrieve names, remember situations, or answer a question. Often, individuals have been told they have Alzheimer's disease; they may or may not remember being told.

It seems unnecessary, even cruel, to give someone false hope. Also, telling someone not to worry never works while he or she is worrying. This is like saying, "Whatever you do, don't scratch your itch!"

The approach with knack is gentle and affirmative. The caregiver validates the person's feeling and offers a practical solution to help the person *remember. It is certainly possible that the* person *will lose the list, or even forget he or she has the list, but the answer is bound to satisfy him or her at that moment.*

★ Hallucinating

A woman with Alzheimer's disease comes up to her son in the family room looking upset, claiming, "There's a big cat in my bedroom. He may hurt me!"

No-Knack Approach

"I bet it's one of those friendly circus animals. They can be really big, but I know how to tame them. Let me get some magic big cat food that I keep in the refrigerator. It will definitely tame him so we can all go to bed later tonight." [moments later] "I just went into the room and we talked and he went back to the circus."

Example of Knack

"You stay here, Mom, and I'll check out the room." [moments later] "Well, Mom, I have some really good news. Everything is okay now!"

Discussion

Sometimes individuals with Alzheimer's disease will hallucinate and see people, animals, or other objects that are not present. They might be mixing up old memories. Seeing an empty yard, for example, may trigger recall of a time when an angry dog really did wander into that yard. They may confuse past and present. What appears to be a hallucination might also be caused by problems in speech. Perhaps the person *means to say a mailman is coming across the front yard, but instead says a madman is crossing the front yard.*

In the above scenario, it is not advisable to embellish the situation to fantastic levels. By taking his mother's worries to such an extreme, the caregiver was not respecting her fears. She may sense his lack of sincerity. Using the knack approach provides a strong indicator that all is well, and should suffice. If the person *continues to talk about animals with concern, the caregiver can use finesse and say, "Oh, Mom, I saw the cat go out the door. It's outside now."*

★ Wanting to Go Home

A wife is perplexed that her husband wants to go home, even though he is at the house he has lived in for 40 years. She cannot imagine why he feels like a stranger in his own home.

No-Knack Approach

[In a high-pitched tone of voice] *"This is your home and has been for 40 years! I can get the deed out of the files to show you. Remember how we slaved to pay for this property?"*

Example of Knack

[Taking his hand and speaking calmly] *"Tell me about home. Let's have some ice cream while we talk about it."*

Discussion

The person may think he is not at home, or he may not be speaking literally; needing to go home may mean getting back to where things make sense again. Confronting him with the facts in an angry tone will make him defensive; he may be convinced he is right because he cannot remember buying the house.

In the above example, the caregiver's interest ("Tell me about home") lets her husband know that she is listening. The open-ended statement allows him to talk awhile, which may help the listener better understand the meaning behind his words. The ice cream can be an excellent distraction.

★ Feeling Sad

Staff at the adult day center notice that one of their favorite participants seems down in the dumps. Normally she enjoys all the activities, including dancing and singing. "I'm very sad today. Nobody loves me anymore," was her reply when asked about her feelings.

No-Knack Approach

"I don't think it's good to feel sorry for yourself. You've got so much to be thankful for. You've got lots of family, including your granddaughter in Taiwan who is visiting you soon, your cousins in Ohio, and your sister in New York. You were happy yesterday; just try to enjoy yourself today."

Example of Knack

"I'm sorry you're feeling blue today. I feel that way now and then too." [pause for her to respond] *"But you know you are my friend and I love you a whole bunch."* [pause for a big hug and time together] *"Your granddaughter will be coming soon. That should be lots of fun."*

Discussion

The no-knack response does not acknowledge the person's feelings. However well-meaning, the staff member presents too much information all at once. Worse, she tries to explain away the problem and argue a different point of view. It is impossible to win an argument with someone with Alzheimer's disease! The final statement, wherein the staff member simply ends by saying, in effect, "Shape up!", probably would not be helpful in any *situation in which someone is feeling blue.*

The approach with knack affirms the person's *feelings of loneliness— not judging, just listening and accepting. The day center staff member admits having similar feelings, which helps the* person *feel that she is not alone, that these feelings happen to all of us. The staff member responds in the present, letting the* person *know that she has one good friend who loves her.*

The staff member also masterfully uses moments of silence to give the person *time to respond. A big hug after a compliment also creates a special connection. Knowing the* person's *life story, the day center staff member is aware that the granddaughter is very special to this participant. She therefore reminds the woman that her granddaughter will be visiting soon, which gives her a good feeling.*

★ Being Overwhelmed by Questions

A family who cares for their grandfather at home finds most of the days pleasant and easy. Yet old friends who are not sensitive to Alzheimer's disease come by several times a week and often ask a string of difficult-to-answer questions. The family notices increased anxiety and restlessness in the grandfather after the friends' visits.

No-Knack Approach

"What did you do today?" "What are your grandchildren up to these days?" "What new songs have you learned recently?"

Example of Knack

"Did you have a good time today?" "How are your grandchildren, Jeremy and Rachel? Are they still on the high school honor roll?" "I bet you enjoy all those old songs you sing so well."

Discussion

The most striking symptom of Alzheimer's disease is memory loss, particularly loss of short-term memory. When we ask someone with dementia questions to which they do not know the answers, it creates feelings of anxiety. It is like the time the teacher called on us and we did not know the answer. We know the feeling very well!

We are prone to ask inappropriate questions that call for a retrieval of facts, forgetting the difficulty this presents to the person. *The first set of questions would prove difficult for most individuals with Alzheimer's disease, causing embarrassment, frustration, and occasionally anger.*

The second set of questions are open-ended and give the person an opportunity to give an acceptable answer of "yes" or "no." In the above example, even if the grandfather does not remember, he can take part in the conversation. It is also possible that an emotional memory is present, so a question phrased "I bet you enjoy . . ." can evoke emotions and meaningful experiences he felt during the day.

The second set of questions again shows the value of using knowledge of the person's life story. In this case, friends can remind him of his grandchildren's names and his love of singing. This type of cueing can also allow the person to recognize names and make a connection, even if he cannot initiate retrieval of the memory.

★ Wanting to Stay Busy

Many older adults remember a time when the workdays were long and the paychecks were small. Despite these conditions, the work ethic was strong. One woman with Alzheimer's disease always wanted to keep busy—clean the house, sweep the porch, and fold clothes. The nursing facility activities staff found themselves growing impatient and exasperated at times because their planned activities did not interest her.

No-Knack Approach

"You don't need to be working all the time. We're going to have fun today. The crafts class starts at 3 o'clock."

Example of Knack

"I need your help. Would you please help me get the room ready for this afternoon? We will be working on gifts to help children. You are my best helper!"

Discussion

Playing was never an acceptable activity for this woman. The work ethic predominated. When the activity is meaningful to her, she will embrace it.

This scenario is a good example of the subtleties of tying one's approach to the person's needs and special issues. The first response, wherein the nursing facility staff member tries to gently cajole her into participating, is certainly friendly and well-intentioned, but it does not respect the person's desire to be productive. The knack approach not only is couched in language the person responds to but also gives her a reason to be involved in what might otherwise seem like a frivolous activity.

★ Coping with Plans Going Awry

The director of an adult day center worked with the astronomy department at the local college to create an ambitious art project involving a mobile of the solar system. Balloons would be covered with pâpier-maché strips and then painted to represent each planet.

On the day of the activity, staff and volunteers gathered together. The director was ready with paper strips and glue. The balloons were colorful, and it was fun blowing them up to different sizes. Suddenly, one program participant batted a balloon in the air, another batted it back, and all the program participants began an extended balloon toss game.

No-Knack Approach

"Let's stop this now! We must get this project finished. Next Tuesday is the day to paint the planets. If we don't get everything done today, we won't be ready. The planets need a week to dry."

Example of Knack

"What fun! Balloons are made for celebrations. I guess the solar system won't change between now and next week if we do the next part of the project later. You know what they say about the best-laid plans!"

Discussion

Often, it is difficult for family members or professionals to let go of their carefully made plans. Yet people with dementia do not share this concern. They live and find joy in the moment.

In this case, the day center director with no knack was frustrated that she would fall behind schedule on her planetary project. The pushing of the participants to move on could create tension and frustration. Would the program participants have gotten any more joy from the completed project than from their spontaneous balloon toss?

The day center director with knack is not afraid to laugh at herself ("the best-laid plans"). In this case, the approach with knack is to take pleasure in the moment, and to complete the pâpier-maché project later. Activities with knack do not focus too much on the end product; the process of the activity is just as important.

★ Coping with Agitation

Many adult day centers have participants who become worried during the day. They may be worried about who will pick them up, or begin to think that they are late for an appointment. Sometimes they are afraid that no one will come and they will be left behind.

No-Knack Approach

"It will be at least 5 hours before your son comes, maybe more! You know he's very busy and sometimes runs late. Just relax!"

Example of Knack

"We are in touch with your son. He'll be here after we sing together. He'll be here soon."

Discussion

The first approach involves several mistakes. First, giving too many details, trying to explain things logically, adds to the confusion and will not be remembered. Second, being too literal ("at least 5 hours") is also a recipe for disaster, particularly because many people with memory loss cannot keep track of the passage of time. Finally, by mentioning that the son is often late, the person may think something is wrong and begin to worry further.

The response with knack is reassuring: "We are in touch with your son," and "he'll be here soon." Note that this stretches the truth somewhat, but still passes the caregiver integrity test. Adult day centers are usually able to reach family members when needed ("we are in touch"), and the word "soon" can be any length of time. In this case, the words are being used in the best interest of the person, to calm fears.

Distraction is also put into play to calm the person. The person's life story suggests an enjoyment of singing, so the mention of that part of the day evokes a smile and good feelings, which replace the anxiety.

★ Confusing Past and Present

Because of the failing memory and confusion that accompanies dementia, often the person will become confused about past and present. A mother might say to her daughter, "I'm waiting for Manuel. I'm sure he'll be home any minute," despite the fact that he is long deceased.

No-Knack Approach

[With exasperation or anger] *"Don't you remember? Father's dead! He's been gone 10 years now. How could you forget such a thing?"*

Example of Knack

"I have such special memories of Dad. It's hard to imagine that he's been gone now for 10 years! Tell me more about Dad. You had a lot of fun going to band concerts together. How about coming over tonight and helping me make dinner? I'll come and get you."

Discussion

One should never ask "Don't you remember?" of a person with Alzheimer's disease. It is a meaningless question with an obvious answer. When the person sometimes thinks that a dead relative is alive, it can be highly upsetting to caregivers. It is important not to overreact, even if painful memories are evoked.

The daughter with knack offered a mild correction that saved face and could help redirect her mother or cue her that Father is gone. She then changed the subject with a request that reminded her mother that she is valued ("Mom . . . how about . . . helping . . .?").

The authors never recommend untruthfully saying that someone is alive. Such a statement oversteps the bounds of caregiver integrity and could backfire in obvious ways.

★ Coping with Inappropriate Sexual Behavior

One of the most upsetting experiences to a caregiver is when the person makes an inappropriate sexual advance. What should happen if a man with Alzheimer's disease makes a sexual advance toward his daughter?

No-Knack Approach

[Angry and outraged] *"You dirty old man! Stop that immediately!"*

Example of Knack

"Daddy, it's Mary, your daughter. Look what I have here—a photograph of Mother. Isn't she pretty?"

Discussion

One quality we strive for in good Alzheimer's care is being calm and collected when problems occur. In this case, the person is not a bad man. He may genuinely be confused about identity. If the person thinks his daughter is his wife, the advance does not seem so out of the ordinary. His confusion could be compounded by the fact that often daughters look like their mothers.

The above response with knack is a sensitive one in so many ways. The daughter clearly identifies herself in one sentence by saying "Daddy, it's Mary, your daughter." Then by showing her father a picture of her mother, she provides further cueing about roles and identities. Finally, the daughter approaches the situation in a calm, nonjudgmental fashion.

It is also important to note that sometimes the label of sexual inappropriateness is applied incorrectly. If a person begins undressing, it might be because he or she is too warm. A man might unzip his pants to go to the bathroom, not to expose himself.

★ Handling Angry Outbursts

Because of the confusion and frustration that can accompany Alzheimer's disease, persons may sometimes become angry and even strike out at caregivers. This can be very upsetting, perhaps even placing the caregiver at risk for injury. However, anger often has an identifiable cause. If the person is being bathed, for example, and becomes angry, it might be out of fear (e.g., fear of being undressed by someone the person may not remember, fear of drowning).

No-Knack Approach

[Rushing up to the *person,* trying to hold him or her down or hold the arms] *"Don't get angry at me! I'm trying to help you! You need to behave!"*

Example of Knack

- Giving the *person* time to cool off

- Distracting the *person*

- Taking the blame ("Dad, I'm sorry I upset you. Will you accept my apology?")

Discussion

The best generals know when to charge ahead and when to retreat. A caregiver with knack never forces the person to do something against his or her will unless absolutely necessary and/or unless all other approaches have failed (e.g., moving a wanderer off a busy street). Caregivers should also consider their own safety and simply leave the house if threatened, call a friend or family member, or call 911.

★ Coping with Repetition

People with Alzheimer's disease often repeat questions or requests. This can, of course, be extremely annoying to caregivers and can cause caregivers to lose their temper. A typical situation might be when the person asks, "When do we have lunch?" over and over again.

No-Knack Approach

"How many times do I have to tell you that we just had lunch! Please be quiet, you're driving me crazy! You just go on and on and on!"

Example of Knack

[Even if lunch was 20 minutes ago] *"Sis, we'll have a meal soon. Here's a piece of fruit to tide you over."*

[Providing a distraction] *"Sis, let's put on those Guy Lombardo records we love so much and see who can still dance the best. Do you remember our first double date?"*

Discussion

Being reprimanded can make the person defensive, even angry, and does little to end the repetition. The approach with knack ("We'll have a meal soon") validates her question. The sister's offer to put on old records and her question about their first double date are wonderful distractions that, it is hoped, will break the pattern of repetitive questions.

★ Taking Other People's Things

Sometimes persons with Alzheimer's disease will pick up something belonging to another because they think it is their property. This error in judgment can create many problems, particularly in a long-term care facility where doors are not locked and staff cannot be everywhere all at once.

No-Knack Approach

"Mrs. Owens, that does not belong to you. Take that back where you found it!"

Example of Knack

"Why, Mrs. Owens, you found my blue coat I had misplaced. Thanks so much for returning it."

Discussion

The first approach, of course, relies on reasoning, which can be short-circuited by Alzheimer's disease. Also, any caregiver is bound to laugh at the thought that Mrs. Owens could successfully take the coat back to where she found it. The object would then not only be misappropriated but misplaced, perhaps never to be found.

The approach with knack is simple and evokes old social graces to thank someone for a favor, in this case finding a "lost coat." The authors recommend that if this approach does not work, staff simply take the coat back while Mrs. Owens is not looking or is involved in another activity. The authors also recommend that day centers, long-term care facilities, and even at-home caregivers continually work to simplify the environment. If caregivers can dispose of unneeded or unused possessions, it can make it easier to keep things in their proper place.

CONCLUSION

Even caregivers with knack will fail on occasion. The nature of Alzheimer's disease is such that there are always good and bad days. An activity or approach may work wonders one day and fail the next. Yet caregivers with knack will always be able to fine-tune their approaches, and approaching problems with knack will never make matters worse. Knack helps us make the best of any situation.

III

The Best Friends Model in Action

Applying the Best Friends model in the areas of communication, activities, the home setting, the day center, and the long-term care facility

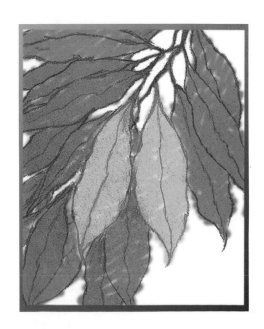

8

The Best Friends Approach to Communication

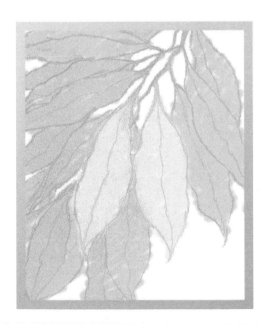

When potential drug therapies for Alzheimer's disease are discussed by families and professionals, the conversation usually revolves around effective treatments for restoring memory. Yet imagine for a moment that a drug was developed that did nothing else for the *person* with Alzheimer's disease but protect speech and communication. This drug could make a big difference in Alzheimer's care. With intact communication skills, the *person* could do the following:

- Express feelings about the disease more clearly and accurately

- Better communicate his or her day-to-day wishes
- Be more responsive to directions and requests
- Share in the decisions
- Be part of evaluating the care he or she receives

This chapter explores the Best Friends model as it is applied to communication between the *person* and his or her caregiver or caregivers. The authors cannot deliver a "magic pill," but many of the ideas offered here will improve communication and make daily interactions productive and meaningful.

The chapter opens with a summary of how the Best Friends model can be applied to communication. A number of brief, scripted scenes that demonstrate good communication are then offered. The chapter concludes with an extended discussion about the importance of looking at the language we use to describe Alzheimer's disease, and how words have an impact on care.

BEST FRIENDS PHILOSOPHY OF COMMUNICATION

The Best Friends model as applied to communication includes the following suggestions for caregivers.

Remember the basics of good communication   The principles of good communication apply to any exchange, even if none of the people involved has Alzheimer's disease. Communication is always enhanced by good eye contact; use of specific, descriptive language; use of appropriate volume and tone; and use of appropriate gestures.

Understand the *person's* desire to communicate   *Persons* with Alzheimer's disease retain the need to communicate long after their vocabulary and language skills diminish. They need to understand and be understood. At the same time, the desire to communicate must be present for the family member or professional. We must employ active listening and work to be there for the *person*.

Make a good first impression   First impressions are everything. We should always identify ourselves, explain our relationship to the *person*, and call the *person* by name. Initiating interactions with a smile and a positive greeting also greatly improves communication. Conversely, taking the *person* by surprise can lead to problems; we must remember that the *person* takes us at face value at each encounter.

Create an environment that facilitates good communication Remember to always consider the world of people with Alzheimer's disease and how it might inhibit communication. They receive messages from everything in their surroundings. Is the house, day center, or facility well-lit, clean, uncluttered, and pleasant, or is it full of potential distractions? Communication is often poor in facilities, for example, as a result of the ambient noises or other distractions in the background. We should try to talk in a relatively quiet place with few distractions. As Rebecca Riley commented (see Chapter 1), "It is difficult to follow conversation with so much noise."

Treat the *person* as an adult We should not use "baby talk" in communication. Simple language can still be adult in nature. We do not need to speak so slowly that it becomes ridiculous. Also, we must be aware of the tendency to use the "royal we." To say things such as, "Let's take *our* medicine now" when only the *person* is taking a pill or "Let's put on *our* pants now" is demeaning and can be confusing to the *person*. He or she might genuinely wonder who will be wearing the pants!

Maintain caregiving integrity The caregiver should not pretend to understand the *person* if he or she does not. If the words cannot be understood, an affirming statement can be made, such as, "Dad, I always enjoy being with you" or "Mom, you usually have all the right ideas." Many *persons* can detect a lack of sincerity; we must not be overly gushy or overly enthused. This can grate on the *person* and others present.

Respond to emotional needs We should try to understand the emotion behind unintelligible words. If the *person* seems upset, we can say, "I'm sorry about that"; when he or she seems happy, we can say, "That must have been great!" If the *person* can articulate concerns or feelings about his or her illness, we can empathize and validate them ("It must be hard to have Alzheimer's disease"). Finally, we should always utilize smiles, handshakes, or hugs to make an emotional connection and provide reassurance.

Remember the importance of nonverbal communication The *person* gets a message from a speaker's tone of voice, posture, volume, and hand gestures. Consider the example of a son telling a funny story to his mother. While telling the story, he laughs, smiles, and has a welcoming posture. His face is animated. Even if his mother does not understand the joke, she picks up his feelings of happiness

THE BEST FRIENDS
PHILOSOPHY OF COMMUNICATION

Remember the basics of good communication

Understand the *person's* desire to communicate

Make a good first impression

Create an environment that facilitates good communication

Treat the *person* as an adult

Maintain caregiving integrity

Respond to emotional needs

Remember the importance of nonverbal communication

Remember that behaviors communicate a message

Do not take the *person* too literally

Employ good timing

Use repetition to facilitate better communication

Do not argue or confront

Screen out troubling messages or news

Speak using positive language

Employ humor in communication

Do most of the work

The Best Friends Approach to Alzheimer's Care, by Virginia Bell and David Troxel.
Copyright © 1997, by Health Professions Press, Inc., Baltimore.

and spirit of fun. Conversely, even positive verbal messages can be undermined if the caregiver is tense or troubled.

Remember that behaviors communicate a message   Early in the disease, the *person* can communicate feelings and problems in words; later, his or her behavior articulates what words cannot. Behaviors such as yelling or striking out can signify that the *person* is in pain. Wandering can suggest boredom. Tears can suggest loneliness and the need for more activity and interaction with other people.

Do not take the *person* too literally   We must recognize that the disease process affects word retrieval and vocabulary. For example, the *person* may think he or she is being clear but may be using the wrong word. He or she may say to a caregiver "Hand me that *glass*" while really meaning "*coffee cup.*"

Employ good timing   We should try to get on the person's wavelength to know when to lend verbal assistance. For example, if by waiting 15 seconds the *person* can complete a sentence, it is always advisable to have patience (even when that 15 seconds seems an eternity) and let the *person* enjoy success. Sometimes when the *person* is trying to express him- or herself, a caregiver can pick out meaningful comments or supply a missing word or phrase. Being a verbal detective can pay off when one makes a connection.

Use repetition to facilitate better communication   Asking a question twice, with additional descriptive cues for greater emphasis, can help the *person* better understand what caregivers are saying: "Mom, hand me that broom [*pointing*] please. Mom, hand me that yellow broom over there [*pointing*]."

Do not argue or confront   The authors wanted to offer a $1 million prize for the individual who could prove to us that he or she had "won" an argument with someone with Alzheimer's disease, but we were overruled by the publisher. We still think our money would have been safe. It is virtually impossible to win an argument with an individual with Alzheimer's disease. Trying to present an argument or to convince the *person* of a particular point of view will lead to frustration and failure. Also, confrontation only causes a *person* to be more defensive.

Screen out troubling messages or news   The *person* has difficulty sorting out information; therefore, it is important to screen out sad, violent, ominous, or controversial messages when possible. Even distressing stories with a happy ending can cause a *person* to worry. For example, if a neighbor tells the *person* that her car was stolen but found a few hours later, the *person* may get stuck in the middle of the story and continue to be concerned about the initial theft.

  Speak using positive language Whenever possible, we should speak to the *person* using positive language. It is better to say "Let's go this way," than "Don't go that way." People with Alzheimer's disease are often proud, and no one likes being told what to do.

  Employ humor in communication Sharing a joke or pun and a corresponding laugh is communication at its finest. It involves bonding and an emotional release. Also, laughter is infectious; we tend to laugh at a joke whether we "get it" or not.

  Do most of the work In good friendships, we compensate for areas of weaknesses in our friends. Because the disease process has an impact on language, we cannot expect the *person* with Alzheimer's disease to do an equal share; we must work harder for good communication.

COMMUNICATING WITH KNACK

The following scripted situations show the Best Friends model as applied to some familiar communication problems. The professionals and family caregivers in these scenarios all show elements of knack in their listening skills, empathy, patience, focus on the present, humor, and attempts to lighten up on life even when things are tough. The caregivers also demonstrate the knack of self-confidence, which the authors hope the Best Friends model will bring out in everyone.

A Wife Asking Her Husband to Take a Specific Action

[*Makes eye contact*] "Lance, come over here." [*Gestures with hands and speaks in pleasant tone*] "Sit with me here on the *sofa*." [*Pats hand on sofa, smiling broadly*] "Come on, come into the living room, right here, this blue sofa is so comfortable. Good." [*Gives a hug*] "I'm glad you're here beside me."

  Note that the caregiver speaks in short, direct sentences. She calls her husband by name, repeats key phrases, and uses gestures and body language effectively. Also, she adds emphasis when she mentions the sofa and then the "blue sofa." Then she gives him an affectionate hug, in a sense rewarding him for coming into the room.

A Day Center Director Using
Descriptive Language to Add Specificity to Directions

[*Hands the participant, Jane, a vase of flowers*] "Jane, would you hold this pretty vase of flowers for me?" [*Gives her time to hold the small vase and admire the flowers*] "Would you put this pretty orange vase [*Gestures*] on that white table [*Points, gives Jane time to locate the table*] over there next to the piano?"

The director showed knack by using descriptive nouns instead of pronouns. She did not vaguely say please put *this* over *there*. Instead, she talked about an orange vase and a white table next to the piano. She also showed patience by handing Jane the vase, letting her admire it, and taking time to let Jane see the table and the piano.

A Day Center Worker Utilizing Elements
of a Life Story to Relate to a Program Participant

[*Gently takes the participant's hand and smiles*] "Good morning, Andrea. I'm your friend, Mary. How are you this morning? I have a surprise for you!" [*Waits for response*] "I remembered that Pablo Picasso is your favorite artist. I brought this book in just for you. You know, I wish everyone had more interest in art like you."

The day center staff member cleverly inserts pieces of Andrea's biography into everyday conversation, making Andrea feel at ease and comfortable with a familiar friend. The fact that the day center staff member has individualized the activity to Andrea's past interests shows good programming. Finally, the last statement, a compliment, always pays dividends.

A Son Coping with His Mother's Accusations

MOTHER: [*Angrily*] You took my purse! Where's my money?

SON: [*Keeps some distance, speaks in a calm voice, looking directly in his mother's eyes*] Mom, it's me, Jeff, your son. You are such a teaser. [*Smiles*] Let me help you. I bet if we look together for a few minutes we'll find that purse.

MOTHER: Jeff, someone took my purse.

SON: Mom, tell me about that purse.

MOTHER: It's my purse.

SON: I think I remember that you had the brown purse out today. Was it the brown purse?

MOTHER: Yes.

SON: Here it is, Mom. You know, I put it in the drawer for safe-keeping. I'm very sorry if I upset you. I won't do it again.

MOTHER: Well, okay. Don't touch it again.

Jeff handles this situation well by keeping his distance initially and letting his mother vent. He introduces himself and then teases his mother a bit, attempting to provide a small distraction. The son says that he had put the purse away for his mother (which may or may not be true). He has the knack of taking the blame for his mother, smoothing over a difficult situation and helping her "save face."

A Sister Trying to Understand Her Brother's Seemingly Incomprehensible Words

GREG: [Looking agitated] Um, that's out. Cold.

LINDA: [Studies Greg's face, sees concern] Greg, is something wrong?

GREG: It's cold. Noise. Cold.

LINDA: It is cold outside. Let's look out the door. Will you help me take a look? [Takes Greg by the hand and gently leads him to the sliding glass door] Brrr, it is cold out there! Show me what you see.

GREG: There was noise.

LINDA: Oh, are you looking at that cat out there? How did Mouser get out? Shall we let him in? He's going to want a warm lap to sit in. I think he likes you, Greg. Let's call him in and go sit by the fire.

Linda demonstrated effective communication by being patient, treating her brother's concerns as real, and piecing together the clues to discover that the cat had indeed gotten out in cold weather. By studying Greg's body language (his face and pacing), she determined that there was a problem and appropriately responded, "Is something wrong?" Perhaps in this case she may also recall that Greg uses the word "noise" when he refers to the cat's "meow." Sometimes the puzzle can be solved.

A Nursing Assistant (CNA) in a Long-Term Care Facility Talking with a Resident Who Is Trying to Make Herself Understood

CNA: [*Passing by Mrs. Arthur in the hallway*] Hello, Mrs. Arthur, I'm Marsha. It's nice to see you again. How is that sweet grandson of yours, Mike?

MRS. ARTHUR: It's just, just there. Do that for me!

CNA: Show me what you mean, Mrs. Arthur.

MRS. ARTHUR: Do that.

CNA: [*Not understanding*] You know, Mrs. Arthur, I enjoy being with you. [*Smiling*] I bet you are very wise about life. I could probably learn a lot from you!

MRS. ARTHUR: [*Smiles and moves on down the hallway*]

Demonstrating knack, Marsha made the best out of a no-win situation. She greeted a resident cheerfully and recalled a fact from her life story to make a connection. Yet Mrs. Arthur's verbal skills have declined to the point that it is difficult to understand what she is saying. In this case, an affirmative statement "I bet you are very wise about life" and then the compliment "I could probably learn a lot from you!" demonstrate respect and affection. Even though the statements stretch the truth a bit, they are said with caregiving integrity.

A Daughter Comforting Her Agitated Mother

MOTHER: [*Pacing back and forth, wringing her hands*]

DAUGHTER: [*Walks up to her mother, smiles, and takes her hands*] Hi, Mom! It's Maureen, your daughter. How are you?

MOTHER: I know who you are!

DAUGHTER: [*Gives her mother a hug, takes her right hand, and gently massages it*] Let me put some of this new lotion on your hands. It smells so nice. [*Rubs in lotion*] Let's walk over and sit down in the family room. [*Pats her mother on the back, guides her mother to the room*]

This example demonstrates that touch in all forms can be a powerful way to communicate. All of us have the need for touch. In this case, Maureen gives her mother a hand massage and a hug. The contact is reassuring and a part of sensitive and loving Alzheimer's care.

A Son Picking Up His Father at the Day Center and Encouraging Him to Take a "Bathroom Break" Before They Drive Home

SON: [*Greets father warmly*] Hey, Dad, how are you doing?

FATHER: No problems.

SON: [*Whispers to him*] Let's stop at the bathroom before we go home.

FATHER: I'm okay.

SON: Okay, let's go. [*Pats his father on the shoulder, smiling, making a hand gesture toward the front door; as they pass by the men's bathroom door, says*] Dad, let's both pop in here for a minute. It's a long way home. [*Successfully leads him into the men's room*]

Sometimes people with Alzheimer's disease will automatically say no to something when they do not quite understand what is being asked of them, or in this case, may not know where the bathroom is. The son showed knack by not embarrassing his father or treating him like a child (he whispered his initial request). Rather than argue, he went ahead and gently coaxed his father again, saying "Let's both pop in." The language used was simple, direct, and active.

CONCLUSION: THE LANGUAGE OF ALZHEIMER'S DISEASE

As noted early in the book, the authors believe that the language used to describe an illness and the people with the illness has an impact on attitudes and affects care. Over the years, we have collected many terms that are used to describe Alzheimer's disease, the *person* with the illness, or the experiences of the caregiver: "the funeral that never ends," "the long goodbye," "the worst of all diseases," "a nightmare," "hopelessness," "powerlessness," "devastating," "tragic," "nothing can be done," "inappropriate behavior," "the loss of self," "victim," "the Alzheimer's person," "a ghost of one's former self," "the lost ones," "the angry stage," "a history of angry behavior," "them and us," "children," "childlike," "just like a 2-year-old," "a stranger," and "a shell of his former self."

Some, perhaps many, of these terms may indeed describe the dark moments all caregivers experience when coping with Alzheimer's disease. Yet the Best Friends model depends on a caregiver's willingness to consider change. The following phrases or words are some that the authors have heard from families who have taken the more positive Best Friends approach: "a challenge," "spending time together," "getting to know my father better," "satisfaction from a job well done," "making new and good friends through support groups," "learning new skills," "facing new roles," "embracing change," "the first time I've ever felt the urge to volunteer for a cause," "becoming an advocate," "learning to ask for help," and "becoming closer to my family by facing this disease together." Families have also told us that Alzheimer's disease has taught them to value the present, to get maximum joy from every day, and to live one day at a time.

One way to change people's attitudes is to change the language families and staff are using to talk about Alzheimer's care. Positive language will refocus a caregiver and his or her way of thinking about the disease.

The authors have already commented in this book about several aspects of language. To recap, we resist the word "victim" because this collapses the *person's* whole being into the disease. We also do not use "patient" or "client" except when a *person* is receiving services from a professional. A *person* is not a patient or client all the time. We do not use "stages of illness," recognizing that stages are arbitrary and lead to false expectations and assumptions.

Careful readers may have noticed several other choices we have made as authors:

1. This book often uses the phrase "caring about" individuals with the disease instead of "caring for" them. It seems more respectful and shifts the focus somewhat away from narrow tasks to a more holistic view of care.

2. We also resist the use of the word "managing" in referring to *persons* with Alzheimer's disease. We do not like this word because the tendency is to think of managing projects and things rather than people. In fact, both authors recall with amusement attending a *1-hour* lecture entitled, "The Complete Management of an Alzheimer's Patient." If only it were that simple!

3. Many readers will have noticed that the book rarely uses the word "respite," which is used in Alzheimer's care to describe the need for caregivers to take a break from the demands of caregiving. It

is also used to describe *services* that provide "respite care," such as in-home programs and adult day services. We strongly recommend every caregiver take a *respite*, or a break, from the demands of caregiving. Yet many programs that are enormously beneficial for the *person* with Alzheimer's disease (such as day centers) are still primarily named "respite programs." We believe this negates the value of these programs for the *person*. The programs are for caregivers *and* the *person,* not one at the exclusion of the other.

4. We also resist phrases such as "caregiver burden," which to us evokes an image of mules carrying their loads up and down mountains. We know that the demands of Alzheimer's care are great, but the Best Friends model is all about learning how to lighten the load.

The good news for the 1990s and beyond is that we are entering a time of great optimism. We need to change the tools we use, such as vocabulary, because new tools will make the lives of caregivers easier. More effective drug treatments, more services, and better long-term care facilities than in the past will be available. The authors hope that new approaches to care, such as the Best Friends model, which would have been unthinkable in the mid-1980s, will provide family and professional caregivers with more skills and confidence to provide excellent care—for their loved ones and themselves.

9

The Best Friends Approach to Activities

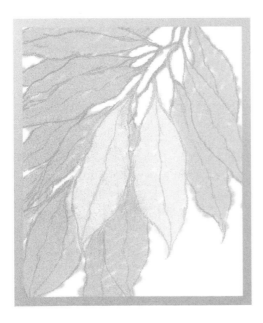

The previous chapters have spoken of the importance of valuing the *person* with Alzheimer's disease as a friend. This philosophy has no better application than in the area of activities. What is friendship if it is not about playing together, working together, and being together?

This chapter begins with a summary of how the Best Friends model can be applied to activities. Next, the purpose of activities in dementia care is examined. Finally, the authors describe some of our favorite activities for people with Alzheimer's disease.

BEST FRIENDS MODEL OF ACTIVITIES

The Best Friends model as applied to activities provides the following suggestions for caregivers and staff (see also p. 132).

A portion of this chapter is adapted from Bell, V. (1995). Creative arts and crafts. In *Activity programming for persons with dementia: A sourcebook.* Chicago: National Alzheimer's Association. Used with permission.

1.   **The art of activities is not in what is done, it is in the doing.** The process of the activity is always more important than the result or end product. If an activity such as folding towels is accompanied by smiles, conversation, friendly gossip, discussion about fabrics and colors, and praise for a job well done, it should not matter if the towels are not folded with perfect edges.

2.   **Activities should be individualized and tap into past interests and skills.** The *person's* life story, as presented in Chapter 6, should be mined for ideas about activities. A *person* who enjoyed playing cards, for example, might not be able to play poker or bridge anymore but might enjoy playing a game with assistance, switching to a simpler game, shuffling the deck, checking the deck to find missing cards, or simply being present and watching others play.

3.   **Activities should be adult in nature.** Activities that are unnecessarily juvenile can provoke frustration, even anger. Some *persons* with Alzheimer's disease respond to dolls or children's toys, but we should not use this fact as an excuse to keep *all* activities at this level.

4.   **Activities should recall a *person's* work-related past.** Many *persons* with Alzheimer's disease enjoy activities that touch on their work-related past, in part because work played an enormous role in their lives. A farmer may still enjoy planting seeds. An artist may want to continue painting. A homemaker may enjoy organizational tasks or a discussion about canning fruits and vegetables.

5.   **Activities should stimulate the five senses (sight, hearing, taste, touch, and smell).** Although some of the senses are diminished by age, many remain strong. The authors have found that the most successful activities stimulate more than one sense. For example, gardening involves touching wet soil, smelling different flowers, hearing the sound of footsteps on autumn leaves, tasting fruit off a tree or a tomato off a vine, and seeing vivid colors in a variety of plants.

6.   **Doing nothing is actually doing something.** Even good friends enjoy quiet times together, perhaps just sitting in the living room listening to music or watching the world go by through a picture window. Sometimes the *person* is content just to be present,

observing others at work, or, depending on his or her level of dementia, the *person* may simply enjoy time alone.

7. **Activities should tap into remaining physical skills.** Many *persons* with Alzheimer's disease remain in remarkably good physical condition. Activities should take advantage of this by including exercise, walking, active chores, or other physical tasks. Many individuals with dementia still have good hand–eye coordination. This skill can be used to advantage in a variety of enjoyable games.

8. **Activities must be initiated by others.** *Persons* with Alzheimer's disease lose the ability to initiate activities. The most well-planned activity will fail if the *person* cannot get started. A retired painter, for example, may still enjoy painting, but he may have to be handed the brush and cued about how to dip the brush in paint and stroke the canvas. Often, this extra push is all that is needed to conduct a successful activity.

9. **Activities should be voluntary.** Most *persons* with dementia will not do something they do not enjoy or find satisfying. No one should be forced to do something against his or her will, particularly in the realm of activities. Of interest is that some caregivers have found that if they begin an activity in front of the *person*, he or she may become interested and then take over the task and continue working happily for a period of time.

10. **Intergenerational activities are especially desirable.** Any staff member of an adult day center with links to a child care center can testify to the fact that intergenerational activities are extremely successful. Both generations benefit from the exchange, and many individuals with dementia enjoy being able to help young people complete a task or project. Again, individual differences must be recognized; for example, W.C. Fields was famous for not liking animals or children!

11. **Activities we think will never work sometimes do.** Many families respond to activity ideas by saying Mother or Father "would never do that." At the same time, staff in day centers and facilities tend to be reluctant to try things that may not succeed. When the authors began work in adult day centers, we were also rather conservative in our activity programming. We soon learned, however, that *persons* with dementia are full of sur-

prises. It is good to question expectations now and then and try new things.

12. **Activities should appeal to the caregiver as well as to the person.** Just as friends tend to seek out activities they both enjoy, activities for *persons* with Alzheimer's disease should be ones that the caregiver, nursing facility staff member, or volunteer also find enjoyable. When this is true, the *person* senses this shared fun, challenge, excitement, or satisfaction.

13. **Personal care is an activity.** Families should recognize that some of the most difficult personal care chores can become more positive when knack is applied. Caregivers can take a few extra moments while helping a *person* bathe or dress to talk about old times, smell a new scented soap, or tell a joke.

14. **Activities can be short.** Sometimes the *person's* attention span makes it difficult for him or her to be involved in an extended activity. Even very brief activities, repeated often, can fill a day. One caregiver would have her father read a number of short poems throughout the day. Another would ask her mother to sweep the kitchen floor often. Even if these activities only last a minute or two, a caregiver can develop a repertoire of short activities that can effectively be put into use during the day.

15. **Activities are everywhere.** With knack, almost everything can become an extended, interesting activity. A simple handshake, for example, can lead to a discussion about fingernail polish, gloves, work done by hand, "lifelines," rings on fingers, engagement rings, weddings, and more. A teapot can be enjoyed for its beauty; discussions can follow about making tea, reading tea leaves, the different flavors of tea, and the Boston Tea Party.

THE PURPOSE OF ACTIVITIES

In our quest to fill the day for *persons* with Alzheimer's disease, we often forget that people do things for a reason. All of us have basic needs that are fulfilled by meaningful activities. In Alzheimer's care, activities meet many purposes or needs.

To Be Productive or to Contribute

Most of us have a need to feel that our lives make a difference to someone or to some community. Maybe we are good at our jobs. Maybe we volunteer in a children's charity. Maybe we are good parents or good friends to others. *Persons* with Alzheimer's disease also retain a desire to help, to feel a part of the world. Activities can help individuals with Alzheimer's disease meet this need to feel competent and useful.

To Experience Successes

Activities can lead to big and small successes. Many children take pride in assembling their first model. A couple who together plant a beautiful garden can be proud of their accomplishment and enjoy the compliments that come from neighbors. *Persons* with Alzheimer's disease have faced many losses. Activities help them rebuild and enjoy new successes.

To Play

Even though many people spend their lives working hard, having fun is still an important part of life for most people. People who have no recreational or fun activities in their lives certainly are missing out on one of life's joys. *Persons* with Alzheimer's disease often retain the ability to enjoy playing, to "lighten up" on life, tease, joke, and engage in activities such as flying a kite. One purpose of activities is to have fun.

To Be with Others

People participate in activities to be with friends, to meet new people, to be part of a club, or simply to feel a part of society. A street festival can include the sights of colorful costumes, the smell of food cooking, and the sounds of enjoyable music. Yet someone might want to feel a sense of belonging, to be with others. Even though *persons* with Alzheimer's disease usually feel more comfortable in smaller group settings, they still have a need for socialization, the need to belong.

To Build Skills

We take part in society and do things to practice what we do well, sharpen old skills, or develop new ones. For example, some *persons*

THE BEST FRIENDS
APPROACH TO ACTIVITIES

The art of activities is not in what is done, it is in the doing.

Activities should be individualized and tap into past interests and skills.

Activities should be adult in nature.

Activities should recall a *person's* work-related past.

Activities should stimulate the five senses (sight, hearing, taste, touch, and smell).

Doing nothing is actually doing something.

Activities should tap into a *person's* remaining physical skills.

Activities must be initiated by others.

Activities should be voluntary.

Intergenerational activities are especially desirable.

Activities we think will never work sometimes do.

Activities should appeal to the caregiver as well as the *person*.

Personal care is an activity.

Activities can be short.

Activities are everywhere.

The Best Friends Approach to Alzheimer's Care, by Virginia Bell and David Troxel.
Copyright © 1997, by Health Professions Press, Inc., Baltimore.

join Toastmasters to practice and improve their public speaking skills. *Persons* with Alzheimer's disease may not necessarily be developing new skills, but activities can help them renew old skills and practice and preserve remaining skills.

To Have a Sense of Control

All of us hope to have some control over our lives. Appropriate activities can help *persons* feel empowered and in charge of their world. For example, some families involve the *person* in simple financial transactions such as signing checks after the checks have been filled out.

To Feel Safe and Secure

All of us have a need for safety and security. If we live in a dangerous neighborhood, fear losing our jobs, or worry about money, these concerns can create stress and strain. *Persons* with Alzheimer's disease have an acute need to feel secure and safe moment to moment. Activities can recall warm feelings associated with past good times and help reassure the *person* that all is well.

To Fill a Religious or Spiritual Need

Although not everyone professes a religious faith, the authors believe that everyone has a *spiritual* life. *Persons* with Alzheimer's disease still may have religious or spiritual needs that can be fulfilled in various ways, including attending religious services, praying, writing poetry, creating art, walking in a forest, or showing compassion for others.

To Experience Growth and Learning

Many people take part in activities to learn more about a particular subject or for human growth. *Persons* with Alzheimer's disease may or may not be able to learn new information, but they still can enjoy the experience of being presented interesting new material. Satisfaction and pleasure come from participation in a learning situation.

SUCCESSFUL ACTIVITIES IN ALZHEIMER'S CARE

When thinking about activities for *persons* with Alzheimer's disease, it can be helpful to think of the activities *we* take part in. What are these activities, and why do we participate in them? What are our favorite things to do? We could think of the activities we have tried in Alzheimer's care. Does the activity fit in with the Best Friends model? Did we enjoy doing the activity with the *person*? Why did the *person* choose to do or not do the activity? What need is that activity filling for the *person*?

Although it is not the authors' intention to provide an extensive list of Alzheimer's care activities, this section outlines types of activities that we have found successful. We encourage readers to use the list as a springboard for their own creativity and, of course, to individualize the activity whenever possible. The reader will note that these activities can be done almost anywhere, at any time, with few materials or little money spent. Activities really are everywhere.

Performing Personal Care

Caregivers with knack work to turn the sometimes-daunting tasks of personal care into activities. The following activities include aspects of personal care:

- Taking a bath can become a bubble bath, with laughter and bubble blowing.
- Dressing can become a fashion show.
- Brushing teeth can become a taste test for a new toothpaste.
- Combing hair can become an opportunity for a quiet sing-along.
- Toileting can be a time to provide extra reassurance.
- Applying makeup can be a time to make fun faces in the mirror.
- Giving a manicure can be a time to compliment the *person*.
- Massaging can create intimacy for a married couple.
- Eating a meal can be a time to ask for an opinion.

Doing Chores

Caregivers with knack help *persons* with Alzheimer's disease feel productive with tasks that mimic the satisfaction many received during their working lives. The caregiver can ask the *person* to help: "Dad, could you help me plant these tulips? You've got such a special touch with plants." This question helps initiate the task and praises the *person's* skills. After the task is done, a compliment can be given: "Dad, thanks to you, we'll have a beautiful garden in spring." The following activities are work-related:

- Gardening can become a fun family activity when someone is squirted with water from the hose.
- Polishing the dining room table can make someone feel useful.
- Folding clothes can keep hand–eye coordination intact.
- Drying dishes can evoke early family memories.
- Raking leaves can be good exercise.
- Cooking can be a chance to smell strong spices.
- Shelling peanuts can evoke the skill of counting.

Being with Pets

Caregivers with knack involve the *person* with friendly family or neighborhood animals when the *person* enjoys such contacts. Pets can provide unqualified love and also provide the *person* with a sense of responsibility when he or she can participate in the care of the animal. The following activities involve pets:

- The singing of a bird can provide an impromptu concert.
- Brushing a dog's fur can be an opportunity to give and receive love.
- Petting a friendly cat results in its soothing purr.
- Feeding ducks can be a highlight of a relaxing, sunny afternoon in the park.
- Schooling tropical fish can provide a kaleidoscope of colors.
- Giving the *person* some responsibility for pet care can make him or her feel needed and can build self-esteem.

Using the Magic of Music

Caregivers with knack know that music is the language of Alzheimer's disease. It is amazing how well many people with dementia enjoy singing a song, listening to music, or playing an instrument. The following activities incorporate music:

- Attending a small church choral concert can be a chance to dress up in fancy clothes.
- Putting on a favorite song can be a wonderful distraction if the *person* is about to become angry.

- Tapping fingers and toes to a pronounced rhythm can provide the *person* with exercise.
- Dancing cheek-to-cheek can be romantic.
- Holding a whistling contest can make everyone laugh.
- Singing familiar songs can reduce anxiety.

Reminiscing

Caregivers with knack encourage reminiscing. It is a basic human need to think about the past and reminisce. People with Alzheimer's disease may have poor short-term memory but early memories are often intact. Sometimes all that is needed to encourage reminiscence is a prop or two and the willingness of the caregiver to ask questions. This type of activity works very well one-on-one or in groups at adult day centers or at facilities. One can reminisce with the following:

- A bottle of perfume, which can evoke memories of a high school prom
- Advertisements of kitchen appliances in a 1950s *Life* magazine
- Old household implements such as a washing board, apple peelers, and a flat iron, which can lead to humorous comparisons between then and now
- Antique farm implements, which can evoke memories of rural life
- Honking the horn of a vintage car, which can bring back memories of a first date

Remembering Old Sayings, Clichés, or Rhymes

Caregivers with knack take advantage of the fact that old sayings, clichés, or rhymes often remain intact in people with Alzheimer's disease. It can be a source of pleasure for them to recall these sayings. It may be even more rewarding when they can teach one of their favorite sayings to others. A group might spend time talking about what an old saying really means. What does "the ox is in the ditch" mean? A farmer might know right away, but "city folk" may struggle. It can also be amusing when a "wrong" answer is given in response to an old phrase; once a day center director told the authors that she asked a group to complete the phrase "The road to hell is paved with _____," and a program participant answered, "committee meetings."

The following examples can be used in activities:

- Flashcards of old sayings could be prepared in a fill-in-the-blank format, creating a pleasurable game for the *person:* "Necessity is the mother of _____."

- Matching rhymes, such as "glad and sad" or "post and toast," can be an activity that can distract a *person* while he or she is being bathed.

- Old sayings can be used in a friendly, teasing way with the *person* to get something done: "A bird in the hand is worth two in the bush."

- Classic poems can be read for enjoyment, and some *persons* might surprise us by recalling them as well.

- Similes relating to animals, such as "loose as a goose" or "naked as a jaybird," can cause the most serious *person* to laugh.

- Reading aloud nursery rhymes can allow the *person* to "teach" something new to children.

Playing Word Games

Caregivers with knack recognize that vocabulary learned long ago can be retrieved through clever word games. These activities tend to work well in group settings or as part of a small family gathering. Most of us can remember the hours that could be filled by these types of games when driving in the car on a family vacation. What makes a game so successful in good Alzheimer's care is that everyone in the room can participate. Because many word games are open-ended, there are almost unlimited right answers. The following ideas for word games can be useful:

- Naming opposites, such as up and down, top and bottom, and right and left, can easily be played at a doctor's office, during a trip, or during other potentially stressful times.

- Listing every word with a certain color, such as Red Sea, red sky, red flag, red-handed, and redhead, can allow *persons* with Alzheimer's disease to participate in group activities.

- Composing a get-well card together can fulfill the need to help others.

- Using Scrabble letters to spell out key words from the *person's* past can be a way to honor the *person's* life story and touch on past achievements.

- Naming state capitals can be a pleasurable memory game in a day center.

Doing Activities with Children

Caregivers with knack know that children can be especially loving and accepting of people with dementia. Intergenerational activities can bring much joy to *persons* in feeling they are helping or teaching young people. The experience can also be valuable to children, who may not have grandparents nearby or living. The possibilities are endless for active (e.g., tossing a ball, painting a picture) or passive (e.g., listening to music, hearing someone read poems) experiences, such as the following:

- Making a Halloween mask together can involve both individuals in a fulfilling art project.

- Reading stories aloud to one another can be an opportunity for praise.

- Walking together can provide exercise and a chance to pick wildflowers.

- Enjoying the festivities surrounding a common birthday: blowing out candles, exchanging presents, singing "Happy Birthday," and eating birthday cake can evoke many smiles and much laughter.

- Being with children can make it acceptable for adults to play childlike games and work simple puzzles.

- Receiving the hugs and kisses children give so freely make the *person* feel loved.

Enjoying Quiet Time

Caregivers with knack design time for quiet reflection or watching the world go by. This kind of quiet time can calm the *person* and help the caregiver recharge his or her batteries. Often, this quiet time can be achieved by identifying daily rituals the *person* has previously enjoyed. The following activities provide quiet moments:

- Visiting the library to flip through all the latest magazines in a quiet, studious atmosphere can often be calming to the *person*.
- Starting a new tradition of afternoon "high tea" and cookies can build a daily ritual.
- Taking a daily walk focuses the *person* on a single task, and can be equally enjoyed by the caregiver.
- Taking a drive down a country road can be a chance to be outdoors.
- Watching hummingbirds sip nectar from flowers can help the *person* connect with nature.

Performing Spiritual Activities

Caregivers with knack learn about the religious or spiritual background of the *person* they care about. Although many nonsectarian programs struggle with fulfilling these needs in such a diverse society, the Best Friends approach calls for individualized activities whenever possible. The following activities can fulfill the *person's* spiritual needs:

- Reading aloud from the Bible or other religious texts can be reassuring.
- Listening to organ music or gospel music can evoke past memories of church activities.
- Praying remains a powerful, symbolic act for many people with dementia.
- Celebrating religious holidays can help a *person* feel connected.
- Involving the *person* in helping a local charity can help him or her feel compassion for others.
- Continuing to attend religious services can help a *person* feel valued.
- Seeing a beautiful sunrise can lift a *person's* spirit and make him or her feel more attuned to the universe.

Recognizing Old Skills

Caregivers with knack take special note of old skills and encourage the *person* to continue to use them as much as possible. Many of these skills were practiced over a lifetime and can be easily cued. Thus, a *person* who played piano well may not be able to learn a simple new song but might, with some cueing (such as humming a few bars), be able to play an old song, even one that is rather complicated. Old skills might include the following:

- Whistling, singing, dancing, or clogging
- Whittling
- Reciting the *Gettysburg Address* or some other memorized speech or poem
- Playing marbles (with a child)
- Carving a corncob pipe
- Cooking fried green tomatoes or another special dish
- Signing one's name with a fountain pen

Creating Arts and Crafts

Arts and crafts provide a wonderful opportunity for *persons* to utilize their remaining strengths and abilities. The nonverbal language of art frees *persons* who have trouble with the complexity of language. Feelings that cannot be expressed in words can often be expressed in art. The sensory exploration of color and texture is stimulating and satisfying.

However, we must remember that arts and crafts projects that are too juvenile might be resisted or rejected by many *persons* who sense that the project is beneath them. All projects should pass one of the Best Friends' "tests" for activities: It should be enjoyed by all involved. In effect, if a project is enjoyed by staff and volunteers or the entire family, the odds are strong it will seem adult enough and be meaningful to the *person*.

People with Alzheimer's disease may enjoy the following creative arts and crafts projects:

- Drawing or painting a memory from childhood, such as a house, school, creek, or forest
- Recognizing familiar paintings seen in an oversized art book
- Using clay to sculpt an animal
- Assembling a mobile from objects gathered on an impromptu scavenger hunt (pinecones, leaves, feathers)
- Creating suncatchers for the windows in a facility

- Filling oranges with dried cloves to give as gifts
- Designing decorations for a holiday party

CONCLUSION

To quote an old song the suggested activities in this chapter represent just "a few of my favorite things." Certainly, there are many more activities that can be done with almost no materials or money and on the spur of the moment. The authors encourage the reader to take on the challenge of doing activities with knack. Many traditional resources or activities fail because they focus on recipes for activities instead of the process of activities. Readers should remember that the Best Friends philosophy is that the secret is not necessarily in what you do—it's in the doing. Life is an activity!

10

The Best Friends Approach at Home

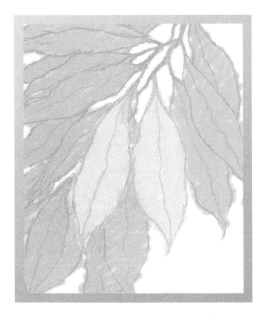

In Alzheimer's care "there's no place like home." Most people with Alzheimer's disease have a strong desire to live in their homes as long as possible. Families share this desire. Paradoxically, the home is often the best of places and the worst of places for Alzheimer's care.

The major benefit of home care is that the care is provided in a familiar place by familiar people. Home care can be economical, particularly if paid in-home caregivers are needed only occasionally. Routines can be maintained. The *person* can enjoy a familiar chair, wear all of his or her favorite clothes, play with the neighborhood cats or dogs, and feel safe and secure. The *person* living at home is still *in* the community and much more likely to see old friends and participate in community events.

The major drawback to home care is that it is most often provided by the spouse, who may alone have to give care that is physically and emotionally stressful. The caregiver may not be able to cope with all of the demands of home care. Other

143

drawbacks to home care include safety concerns when unfamiliar health care providers come into the home, the lack of services in some communities, transportation problems in rural areas, and the expense of in-home care when more help is needed. For example, 24-hour in-home care is almost always more expensive than institutional care.

This chapter examines how the Best Friends model can be incorporated into home care in order to help caregivers achieve their oft-stated goal of keeping their family members at home as long as possible and as long as is advisable. The first section describes the Best Friends model as it can be applied to the home setting. The next section examines various issues surrounding home care, including the changing demographics of the family, living alone, the rising cost of care, conducting activities in the home, asking for help, and coping with changing family roles and relationships. Finally, there is a brief section on the types of services that can help home-based caregivers. (Chapter 12, which covers long-term care facilities, includes a section on *when* to make a placement, valuable for home-based caregivers struggling to make this decision.)

A note about how the authors define home care: We have written this chapter for people caring for a spouse in the family home, adult children trying to help parents remain at home, a neighbor informally helping an older adult who lives alone, or for any individual in a situation in which care is provided in a home setting.

THE BEST FRIENDS MODEL IN THE HOME

The line from John Donne's *Devotions Upon Emergent Occasions*, "No man is an island," is an important starting point for families caring for someone with Alzheimer's disease at home. Caregivers who isolate themselves are bound to have more difficult care-providing experiences. Families should embrace the following elements of the Best Friends philosophy that apply to in-home care:

1. **Be open with others about the family situation.** The stigma of Alzheimer's disease is diminishing rapidly. Families attending support groups for the first time often are surprised to find people they know, maybe even neighbors. Being open about a loved one's diagnosis and the family's goals to provide home care can allow friends and neighbors to offer assistance and can lead to an expanded support network.

2. **Make an honest assessment.** When providing home care, it is important to have realistic expectations about the *person* and oneself, and to review these expectations often. Caregivers should think about their own health, their own attitudes about caregiving, their financial resources, and their coping skills. The *person's* abilities and situation should be assessed, as detailed in Chapter 3. Also, caregivers should assess their home setting, looking at their houses and considering issues of home safety, including locks, fencing, and lighting. In addition, they should think about the community services (or lack thereof) that can be a partner in caregiving.

3. **Continue to be part of the community.** It is important to let the *person* enjoy routines as long as possible. Going out for breakfast, enjoying a concert in the park, taking a daily drive, going to a worship service, and doing other things outside of the house are all part of life and should be incorporated into the *person's* routine whenever possible. Caregivers should remember the knack of creativity. If the regular worship service is too crowded for the *person* to enjoy, a different service can be attended. Going out to breakfast at 10 A.M. instead of the busy hours from 7 A.M. to 9 A.M. may be more enjoyable. The restaurant staff can be informed of the *person's* diagnosis so they can greet him or her with a warm smile and provide extra service when needed.

4. **Recognize that past patterns and rituals may change.** Many homemakers try to hold on to all of their standards of how a household should run. This is not possible when a member of the household has dementia. Caregivers should remember the knack of flexibility. A homemaker who is always organized and keeps an immaculate house must learn to accept that the *person* is unlikely to hang up his or her clothes or put away the dishes. It is very hard for some caregivers to accept, but part of dealing with Alzheimer's disease is letting go of perfection. One caregiver told the authors that she began to think of her husband as a welcome "house guest." She realized that she was often short-tempered with her children when they did not live up to her standards, but she would never say to a guest, "Shut that cabinet after you open it!" or "Can't you pick up after yourself?" This

recasting of relationships was very creative, another element of knack.

5. **Simplify the environment whenever possible.** Part of the knack of good Alzheimer's care in the home is to simplify the household. If the *person* struggles with decisions about what to wear, he or she should not have a closet full of outfits from which to choose. If the *person* has poor judgment, valuable, breakable collectibles should be locked away. If the *person* is unsteady on his or her feet, furniture, area rugs, or objects that clutter pathways and could lead to injury should be removed.

6. **Value and focus on the present.** The authors encourage caregivers to try to let go of past differences. Often, as a result of the disease process, the *person* has forgotten these bad times. Caregivers should focus on providing the maximum in quality of life out of each day, for themselves and for the *person* they care about.

7. **Incorporate the Alzheimer's Disease Bill of Rights into the goals for care.** Caregivers should use the Alzheimer's Disease Bill of Rights as a source of ideas for activities and goal setting (see Chapter 4). For example, the Alzheimer's Disease Bill of Rights suggests that caregivers provide activities that stimulate the senses, allow the *person* time outdoors, and create opportunities to give plenty of hugs.

8. **Turn the *person's* busy work into real work whenever possible.** Because there are many chores associated with running a household, the caregiver should try to involve the *person* in constructive activities whenever possible. If the *person* can still dust a table, sweep a floor, rake leaves, or help in some other capacity, he or she should be allowed to do so.

9. **Enjoy quiet moments and simple pleasures.** Quiet moments of togetherness, such as a morning cup of coffee (decaffeinated!) or listening to music, can be enjoyed by both the *person* and the caregiver. Anything can be an activity! If shrubs must be trimmed, the time can be used as a chance to observe nature or ask the *person* for his or her opinion of how the yard looks.

10. **Do not wait too long to take advantage of community resources and services.** Families often wait and wait and wait to use needed services. Finally, when the *person* has deteriorated

beyond the family's ability to provide him or her with good care, they seek help. Family members then find themselves stymied by waiting lists and forced to make important decisions under pressure. Caregivers should remember the knack of planning ahead.

Issues Affecting Home Care

The Changing Family

The traditional nuclear family as portrayed in 1950s television programs, such as *Leave It to Beaver*, is no longer the norm. In most cases both spouses work, and it is no longer assumed that a wife, a daughter, or a daughter-in-law will take on all the duties of caring for older family members.

The Bureau of the Census defines a family as "two or more persons related by birth, marriage, or adoption who reside in the same household." Yet the reality of families in the 1990s is captured by a national poll that found that most Americans conceive of family as "a group of people who love and care for each other." These groups of people are changing the face of home care. The groups include traditional families with a wage-earning father and homemaker mother; reversed-role families with a homemaking father; families headed by a dual-career mother and father; families in which grandparents are raising grandchildren as a result of parental incapacity or death; families with stepchildren; single-parent families created by abandonment, divorce, death, unplanned pregnancies, or choice; gay and lesbian households; families that postpone childbirth past traditional childbearing age; "sandwich generation" families, in which parents care for young children and older family members at the same time; multi- even four-generation households; unmarried domestic partners; and many examples of older adults living together who may not marry.

These dramatic changes in family life have produced new challenges for providers of care. As an illustration, we may consider the significance of just two of the above examples—grandparents raising children and women postponing childbirth. These trends could lead to more teenagers being responsible for caring for older adults. Will current family support groups, for example, meet their needs?

The authors have worked with primary caregivers whose ages

ranged from the teens to the 90s. The caregivers vary in attitudes, experience, coping skills, and values. They come from widely differing family, social, and community backgrounds. Every caregiving situation is somewhat different, and all have positive and negative attributes.

Long-Distance Caregiving

Families in the 1990s are far-flung. Older adults often live alone and far from their children. This trend, for example, has fueled the growth of the profession of geriatric care managers, which is examined later in this chapter. Children who see their parents occasionally may not always notice subtle changes in a parent's behavior at the onset of Alzheimer's disease. Significant problems such as financial or physical abuse can arise before the family can act.

Older Adults Living Alone

Although this chapter is written primarily for family caregivers, there are many informal caregivers helping an older neighbor or friend who may live alone. This trend is growing because families are getting smaller; often, there is no large, extended family to provide care. Sometimes family members are estranged. Service providers face significant challenges in providing care to individuals who want to live at home, but should not. How do we persuade them to accept help?

Rising Cost of Care

One significant problem facing families is the enormous rise in health care costs. The days of families finding a student to live in and help out in exchange for room and board are past. The costs of caring for someone with Alzheimer's disease can threaten a family's financial security, perhaps even wipe out the "nest egg" aging parents had hoped to leave to children and grandchildren.

Medicaid coverage is available for long-term care when a *person* qualifies for the benefit. Unfortunately, government financial support for people caring for family members at home is limited.

Although the Best Friends model cannot solve the aforementioned problems, it does encourage caregivers to take advantage of available resources and to plan ahead. Doing so will help caregivers avoid financial difficulties.

Training Issues in the Home

Home care is an area in which one does not usually think of training issues, but the authors encourage families to consider three specific issues that can improve home care.

Training Yourself

Families should make a commitment to teach themselves as much as possible about Alzheimer's disease and good Alzheimer's care. Many chapters of the Alzheimer's Association and other groups sponsor excellent workshops and conferences throughout the year. These meetings should be attended whenever possible and other family members should be encouraged to attend.

Training In-Home Caregivers

Because most home health care providers have had limited training in Alzheimer's care, it is vital for families to help fill in gaps in knowledge and to develop strategies to teach home health care providers more about good care. Families can use the Best Friends model as a simple curriculum for these caregivers, as follows:

1. Train in-home caregivers in the basics of Alzheimer's disease and teach them to understand the experience of Alzheimer's disease. These goals can be accomplished by sharing some of the sections of this book with in-home caregivers, attending workshops with them, or showing a video borrowed from an Alzheimer's Association chapter.

2. Share the material on friendship covered in Chapter 5 with caregivers. Ask them what qualities of friendship they value. Ask them to think about their own best friends and the qualities that make the friendships good.

3. Teach by doing: Show in-home care providers the strategies and steps that have worked best.

4. Review the Alzheimer's Disease Bill of Rights (see Chapter 4) with in-home caregivers and use each point as a basis to talk about the family's goals for home care.

5. Explain to in-home caregivers what "knack" means. Ask them to think about and identify friends or co-workers who have knack. Talk about why they feel this is the case.

In a perfect world, all in-home care providers would come to the job (and to the home) well-trained in dementia care and full of knack. Unfortunately, this is rare. Taking even a few hours to talk about good care with paid caregivers is a good investment.

Training Friends and Family

Friends and family members not in the immediate caregiving circle may not always understand what Alzheimer's disease is about. They may have inaccurate preconceived ideas, they may be fearful about visiting, and they may be uncertain what to say. Many of these individuals would not appreciate caregiver attempts to "train" them about dementia, but they may appreciate receiving an occasional brochure, a clipping from a newspaper or magazine, or an invitation to a support group or conference. It is in the caregiver's interest to have friends and family who are familiar with dementia; people who are familiar with dementia can offer more sensitive emotional support, or even help with caregiving if they feel comfortable with the situation. If nothing else, a copy of the Alzheimer's Disease Bill of Rights will provide friends and family members with much information about what constitutes good care.

Conducting Activities in the Home

Caregivers often struggle to keep their loved ones involved in daily life. Many *persons* have led a full, active life; therefore, they need to remain busy in order to maximize remaining abilities. Boredom is not good for anyone, especially for *someone* with Alzheimer's disease. By now, the reader should be comfortable with the Best Friends model. There is also an art to doing things in the home. Home activities encompass the knack of creativity, flexibility, patience, and the ability to make something out of nothing.

The Best Friends model encourages caregivers to think about the process of the activities instead of the result. The authors always resist comparing people with Alzheimer's disease to children, but one example that is particularly meaningful is the following: A father might teach his young son or daughter how to make a bird feeder. The teaching process may involve reading books about bird feeders, walking through the neighborhood to see examples, studying the birds in the backyard to get a feel for the proper size birdhouse, drawing up a simple plan, choosing the wood, cutting the wood, choosing paint colors, and assembling the finished product. Another part of the process might involve studying the best placement in the yard and then thinking of sly solutions to keep the family cat from feasting on the birds and keep the squirrels away from the seeds.

In this family activity, what is more important, how the bird feeder ultimately looks and works, or the learning process that went along with the project? Ultimately, the shared experiences, the father–child bonding, and the time spent together are more important than whether the dimensions of the feeder are perfect.

The authors adopt a similar attitude toward conducting activities in the home. Does it matter if a shoe is perfectly shined if it has kept the *person* productively busy for an hour? Does every leaf in the yard need to be raked? Does it matter if a game is played exactly according to the rules?

"Home Activities" (see p. 152) lists some activities that can be done at home, as well as some general points about activities in the home.

It is also very smart for caregivers who find ideas that work to use them often, building them into daily routines. Thus, if the *person* thrives on taking a ride in the car, try to build it into the daily schedule at roughly the same time. Other families have discovered that a daily teatime or cocktail hour (with nonalcoholic wine or beer) can be a pleasant ritual. However, caregivers should remember that in good Alzheimer's care, a routine is good but a *rigid* routine is bad.

The authors also encourage families not to be afraid to try new things. If a *person* feels secure, if he or she is receiving warm, comfortable feelings and words from the caregiver, it can be amazing how well an unusual activity will work. Taking a loved one to a professional baseball game might turn out to be an enormous success, but the caregiver should be prepared to leave after a few innings if the experience becomes overwhelming. Other activities that can be done in the community are listed in "Community Activities" (see p. 153).

Asking for Help

Activities do not always have to be arranged and carried out solely by the caregiver. As hard as it is to ask for help from friends and family members, part of the knack of good Alzheimer's care is not trying to do it all on one's own.

It used to be common for neighbors to borrow a cup of sugar or

HOME ACTIVITIES

Kitchen

Bake cookies
Clean the windows
Share a cup of coffee
Plant spring bulbs
Enjoy the morning paper

Family room

Play tic-tac-toe
Watch a nature video
Pet the dog or cat
Sit by the fire
Mend a favorite afghan

Patio

Blow bubbles
Bird watch
Garden in containers
Sweep the patio
Have an impromptu picnic

Living room

Sing songs around the piano
Look at old photographs
Read a story aloud
Invite a friend in for a chat
Display a childhood toy

Bedroom

Fold laundry
Display family pictures
Hang awards and plaques
Rearrange drawers
Admire a jewelry collection

Yard

Watch the squirrels
Visit a neighbor
Work in the garden
Watch for the mail carrier
Fly a kite

In general, home activities should:

Be constructive when possible, such as helping with a chore or task

Be activities, such as baking, sewing, or watching scenes from a favorite old movie on video, that the caregiver also finds enjoyable

Encourage reminiscence

Stimulate the five senses (taste, touch, scent, hearing, and sight)

Encourage autonomy

Fulfill the *person's* need to be helpful and to make a contribution

Encourage physical exercise or work

Preserve dignity

The Best Friends Approach to Alzheimer's Care, by Virginia Bell and David Troxel.
Copyright © 1997, by Health Professions Press, Inc., Baltimore.

COMMUNITY ACTIVITIES

Go for a drive

Sit on a park bench

Attend church or synagogue

Visit your favorite ice cream parlor

Practice golf at the driving range

Enjoy a farmer's market

Go to a flea market

Walk in the mall

Visit a friend

Go to the zoo

Attend an exhibit at an art museum

Swim in the neighborhood pool

Run errands together

Attend a granddaughter's soccer game

Attend a class together

Get to know other couples who are coping
   with Alzheimer's disease

The Best Friends Approach to Alzheimer's Care, by Virginia Bell and David Troxel.
Copyright © 1997, by Health Professions Press, Inc., Baltimore.

help each other with occasional favors. This custom has gone out of style in most communities. Some neighbors do not even know each other. In this environment, caregivers often are loathe to ask for help, even from close friends and family members. One caregiver (the adult child of a parent with Alzheimer's disease) summed up her situation as, "My neighbors and friends are so busy. I hate to ask them for anything. Anyway, I don't think I should have to ask my family for help. They should know I need it."

But does the family know? During a family conference, several family members made the following comments about their sister: "I just don't know what she needs. She doesn't tell me." "I don't think she really wants my help." Another family member said, "I did take care of Dad once for a weekend and Sis seemed rather critical of the job I did." The difficulties in this situation range from poor communication to the caregiver's reluctance to ask for help, as if somehow asking for help is admitting failure. Asking for help is tough, but the most successful caregivers use every resource they can. No caregiver is an island.

The following lists some suggestions on how to ask friends and family for help:

- Be specific in requests: "Son, I would like you to come for Dad's birthday. Please make it a priority if you can." A neighbor who wants to help might be asked to pick up some groceries occasionally.

- Do not assume family members should know one's needs. Express needs to family members so they have a chance to help in their own way. Consider putting requests in writing to family and friends to better communicate feelings and wishes.

- Recognize that family members are also coping with denial and other emotions about their loved one's illness. Give them time to cope.

- Recognize that some family members have the capacity to do more than others.

- Do not assume that requests for help will be a burden to family members. They often want to help and gain satisfaction from returning love and care.

- Try not to be overly critical or judgmental about others' attempts to provide help or support. Many times people are well-intentioned even when their contribution has, in fact, been minimal. Giving them a second chance might encourage them to become involved further.

* Remember the biblical saying, "It is more blessed to give than to receive." Many friends or neighbors who are offering to help may want the pleasure and satisfaction of giving the gift of time or help.

Sometimes a caregiver becomes so immersed in the role that he or she rejects help from other family members while bemoaning the fact that he or she is the only one doing the work. There are only two losers in martyrdom. The caregiver begins to lose ties with friends and family and strain other relationships. He or she also tends to shut the *person* off from services, friends, and family who can provide important and loving care. In these cases, the authors recommend convening a family meeting to express feelings and iron out roles for every member. An outside facilitator can sometimes assure that good listening and hearing are taking place.

Conversely, caregivers may repeatedly ask family members for help and the request falls on deaf ears. This sort of rejection can be a bitter pill for a parent or sibling. These disappointments are a part of life and, ultimately, the family member who has chosen not to help will have to come to terms with his or her decision. Meanwhile, caregivers should focus on and enjoy the positive relationships with family members who are being supportive.

COMMUNITY RESOURCES FOR HOME-BASED CARE

One theme of this book is that being a Best Friend to a *person* with Alzheimer's disease means trying one's best to surround him or her with good care. For most families, good care in the home necessitates using community services.

Many community services can be helpful to people providing care at home. Because such services, and even the names of these services, vary greatly by community, this section refers to them only by a generic name. Appendix A lists national agencies that can provide information and referral or other assistance to professional and family caregivers.

The following services can be lifesavers for families caring for individuals with Alzheimer's disease in the home.

Alzheimer's Association

The over 200 chapters of the Alzheimer's Association should be the first resource to which families turn for help. Association chapters provide nonbiased information and referral. They offer many services in the areas of education, patient and family services, advocacy, and support for research. Their chapter-sponsored support groups, newsletters, Safe Return program, and telephone Help-Lines (some of which are open 24 hours a day) are particularly helpful. Many chapters offer a sophisticated array of services, yet even the smallest chapters provide caring, dedicated staff and volunteers who will do their best to help.

Adult Day Services

As mentioned in Chapter 11, the authors are strong advocates of adult day services, which we consider a "treatment" for Alzheimer's disease. Adult day centers provide supervision and enrichment of older people while giving care providers a break. Center staff can also help families link up with other community services. Some centers are dementia specific, whereas others combine frail older people and people with cognitive losses. Readers who have a day center in their area should pay a visit today!

Area Agencies on Aging

Area Agencies on Aging are the conduits for many federal, state, and local funds that go to programs for older adults in the community. They also advocate for improved services for older adults and often offer a comprehensive array of services, including legal services, information and referral services, and care management programs.

Church and Interfaith Volunteer Programs

Many churches have responded to the aging of the American population with services specifically aimed at older adults. For example, the number of parish nurses has increased. Also, churches sometimes use volunteers who travel to a caregiver's home to provide respite. Readers who are members of a church can go there for counseling and support.

Elder Abuse Intervention Services

Elder abuse intervention programs investigate charges of elder mistreatment, including violence or neglect. Notably, these programs also investigate financial abuse or exploitation, a growing problem.

Friendly Visiting

Some government and private organizations have friendly visiting programs in which paid workers or volunteers make regular visits to a home-bound *person* to spend time with him or her and make certain all is well.

Geriatric Assessment Programs/Nurses

Some agencies employ teams that make home visits to assess the health of an older adult and make recommendations for needed services. The agency may charge for the assessment.

Geriatric Care Managers

Geriatric care management is a relatively new health care industry comprised of individuals who will help set up services, handle bill paying, and provide care advice for an hourly fee. The typical care manager is a registered nurse or social worker. Caregivers should select companies or individuals who are members of the National Association of Professional Geriatric Care Managers, but should check references—this is an unregulated industry. Geriatric care management can be particularly valuable for long-distance caregivers who want a responsible party to be able to "look in on Mom (or Dad)," or for working caregivers who can afford to pay someone to help develop a care plan. These managers can also help with hiring in-home help and with nursing facility placement.

Home Health Aides

Home health aides can handle nursing-related tasks such as administering medications, and can also help with bathing, dressing, and other personal care tasks.

Homemaker Services

Homemaker services programs help older adults with household services such as laundry, shopping, cooking, and cleaning. Homemakers can also take care of personal tasks such as bathing, dressing, hair care, eating, and other personal care activities.

Nutritional Programs and Home-Delivered Meals

Many communities have "nutrition sites" where older adults can go for a free or low-cost meal. Meals on Wheels food delivery services may be available for older adults who are homebound.

Overnight, Weekend, or Short-Term Respite Programs

Some nursing facilities or adult day centers offer overnight, weekend, or short-term care. This type of care can be invaluable to caregivers who need some time away for a family visit, in an emergency, or just to take a vacation.

Senior Centers

Senior centers are often the focal point for older adult services and activities. For example, at a senior center a family might find a helpful booklet on how to hire in-home help. Families should visit the centers to learn about their programs and to see if any of the activities might be appropriate for the *person*.

Senior Peer Counseling

Some communities have developed peer counseling programs that can send a trained volunteer to an individual's home to offer guidance and counseling. Many family members find counseling services to be invaluable as a way of coping with the changes in their life, grief issues, and family conflict.

University-Based Memory Disorder Clinics

Many universities have developed specialized memory disorder clinics as part of an overall research effort. These clinics often have a team approach to care, with physicians, nurses, social workers, and neuropsychologists operating as part of a coordinated effort to make a diagnosis and provide continuing support to families. The clinics also take part in experimental drug studies.

Visiting Nurse Associations/Home Health Agencies

Many visiting nurse associations/home health agencies (nonprofit and for-profit) can come to the *person's* home to assess his or her physical health or to provide ongoing services. Services are often covered by Medicare and private insurance. Many home health agencies schedule an initial visit to make an assessment of the *person* and to open a case file. Having this case file can be a lifesaver in an emergency, such as a caregiver's illness. The agency can then initiate services and will already have family contact numbers, doctors' names, and medical information.

CONCLUSION

With in-home care, the art of recasting one's relationship to the *person* with Alzheimer's disease becomes very important. As noted in Chapter 5, relationships change. Thinking of ourselves as a Best Friend to the *person* we care about can help us develop a more relaxed, natural caring style and can give us tools to bring out the best in the *person*.

Contrary to many caregivers' expectations, home care often fails not because of the *person's* worsening health but because the caregiver becomes too strained, too fatigued. If the time comes to make a placement, caregivers can take pride in the fact that they have done their best.

If, as caregivers, we can learn the Best Friends model and approach care with knack, the odds are much stronger that we will be able to keep the *person* we care about at home longer.

II

The Best Friends Approach in Adult Day Services

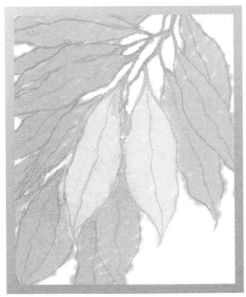

The increase in adult day services is one of the most encouraging trends in the national effort to help *persons* with Alzheimer's disease and their families. For participants, these services can provide a day spent with friends enjoying creative activities in a safe, secure, and stimulating environment. For caregivers, these programs offer an opportunity to continue gainful employment or to take a break from the demands of care.

When the authors began their work in Alzheimer's disease in the early 1980s, most people thought of adult day centers strictly as a respite service for caregivers. It was quickly noticed, however, that the centers were doing much more than helping the caregiver—they were helping the *person* with Alzheimer's disease. Caregivers reported that their loved ones seemed happier, exhibited fewer troublesome behaviors, and slept through the night more frequently. One skeptical neurologist even finally confessed to us in the following words about adult day center care: "I have to admit it—it *is* the treatment for Alzheimer's."

Yet even with the tremendous praise that has been heaped on adult day centers by professionals and family members, this relatively new industry faces many challenges, including the following:

- Public awareness of adult day centers is still rather limited.

- Families do not rush to use services even when it appears that such services would provide many benefits.

- Volunteers are always needed.

- Funding remains a challenge because most centers rely on private and public subsidies to continue operating.

- Adult day centers continue to seek innovative training programs for staff and volunteers.

- Staff struggle to keep activities fresh and meaningful to program participants.

This chapter suggests that many of these challenges can be met when day centers adopt the Best Friends model. The model helps centers develop a guiding philosophy of care, encompassing the themes spelled out in the Alzheimer's Disease Bill of Rights. The model also provides centers with a framework for activities, volunteer recruitment, staff training, and family relations.

Various models of day services are available in the United States, including a health or medical model that offers medical supervision or rehabilitation and a day treatment model that addresses psychiatric disorders. Social adult day services offer supervision, socialization, and life enrichment. The concepts examined in this chapter are broadly applicable to any type of adult day center. The chapter is written primarily for staff and volunteers of adult day centers, although the conclusion has some special words for families considering or using day services.

A note about terminology: These programs have many names, including "adult day care," "day care," and "Alzheimer's day program." In some communities, a day center may have a club-like name (e.g., Sunshine Terrace in Logan, Utah, or Cedar Acres in Janesville, Wisconsin). In this chapter the authors use the terms "adult day centers," "adult day services," or simply "centers" to describe these programs.

We avoid "day care" because the perception of many people is that day care is primarily for children.

THE ADULT DAY CENTER MOVEMENT

Adult day services is a growth industry in the United States. Whereas there were only 20 centers in 1969, by 1996 there were over 3,000 adult day centers, according to the National Adult Day Services Association, part of the National Council on Aging. With the changing demographics of the U.S. population, it can be predicted that early in the 21st century there will be more adult day centers in operation than child care centers.

These centers, many of which are specifically for people with dementia, provide supervised activities and care during the day for frail older adults and people with dementia. Some centers also serve a mixed population of individuals with developmental disabilities, head injury, or other special needs.

Adult day services can be one of the best values in long-term care. Although daily costs vary, the maximum charge is often between $40 and $50/day, roughly $5 to $6/hour. In-home care easily can be double or triple that hourly amount. Also, many of these programs receive subsidies and therefore are likely to have sliding fee scales.

THE BEST FRIENDS MODEL AS APPLIED IN ADULT DAY CENTERS

Day centers around the United States do an amazing job of relating to their participants with Alzheimer's disease. Many centers also serve people through much of the continuum of Alzheimer's disease. What is their secret? Why do their programs tend to be so successful?

Much of their success stems from the fact that day center programs bring out the "social graces" of their program participants. The best programs create a joyful, fun atmosphere or milieu; participants might imagine that they are at a party or at a club. When we are at a special event or around company, we tend to be on our best behavior. It is as if all the manners our parents drilled into us are recalled.

Day centers should consider adopting the Best Friends model of Alzheimer's care in part because it reinforces these social graces. Day centers seeking to adopt this model should mine this entire text for ideas, but the following are some facets of the model that are particularly important:

1. **Volunteers and staff members can become Best Friends to a program participant.** Adult day centers are encouraged to recruit volunteers or assign certain staff members to be a Best Friend to a participant who needs one-on-one attention. If a staff member works regularly with this participant, he or she can learn the most effective ways to bring out the best in the *person* and prevent problems.

2. **The life story can easily be incorporated into care.** Because day centers tend to be small programs, staff generally are able to learn each participant's life story very well (of course, the authors hope that large programs achieve the same goal). Staff should be encouraged to use the life story throughout the day in various activities.

3. **Adult day services can implement meaningful activities.** The philosophy of activities described in this book can easily be adopted by day centers seeking to improve their current programs. Two of the most important Best Friends rules for activities are that the process is more important than the result and that activities are everywhere.

4. **Adult day centers usually have dementia-friendly staff–participant ratios.** Through intensive staffing and use of volunteers, many day programs can offer a high staff–participant ratio. This high ratio allows day programs to individualize care better. Thus, if the *person* is having a bad day and needs someone to take him or her for a walk, staff are available to meet this need. Day centers really can help the *person* find a friend.

STAFF AND VOLUNTEER TRAINING

The Best Friends model can help invigorate training of staff and volunteers. First, centers should recruit staff members who have the potential to develop knack; everything else can follow. Day centers should look for staff in unconventional places; one day center director facetiously remarked to the authors that beauticians and bartenders would make ideal staff members because they are people oriented.

People with knack can always be trained later in the basics of Alzheimer's care.

All staff should be asked to think about their own best friends and the qualities that make these friendships good. Staff can discuss how administrators of the adult day center program can take the best qualities of good friendship and use them in setting up a program philosophy. The idea of treating *persons* with Alzheimer's disease as friends is a simple one. Every staff member can learn and put this idea into his or her own words and thoughts.

Ideas for training staff based on the Best Friends model include the following:

1. *All* staff should be trained in the basics of Alzheimer's disease and should be taught to understand the experience of Alzheimer's disease through lectures, talks with family members, videos, and on-site experience.

2. Role-playing can be an effective learning device, but in day centers with small groups it is best for the key staff member to demonstrate pointers or concepts in the program. For example, it is easy to show a new staff member how to greet participants and their families in the morning. Instead of playing a role, every staff member can be a role model.

3. Staff should be encouraged to think about the knack of good Alzheimer's care. A weekly award can be given to the staff member who best demonstrates knack in a particular situation.

4. Staff should review the Alzheimer's Disease Bill of Rights (Chapter 4). Copies can be posted in conspicuous places to let families, participants, and staff know that these are the center's goals.

5. As is examined in Chapter 12, the Best Friends model is multicultural because friendship is a universally understood concept. Thus, the concepts are easy to explain and demonstrate to staff and volunteers from different cultures.

6. Volunteers should have training equal to that for staff to ensure that they have the skills they need to operate in the program.

ACTIVITIES IN ADULT DAY CENTERS

The fundamentals of day center programs are that the *person* leaves his or her house, gathers with others, and does things. This sounds just like what all of us do when we decide to get together with friends. This section builds on the activities discussed in Chapter 9 and offers pointers on how the Best Friends model translates into activities in the day center setting.

Application of the Best Friends Model

The Best Friends model as applied in day center activities includes the following concepts.

Taking Advantage of the Group Milieu

Much can be done with participants sitting in circles, including exercise, group discussions, and games. The power of a circle is that it can shut out distractions and focus group members on one another. Key volunteers and staff members should sit next to participants who need additional prompting or assistance. Staff should remember the knack of "saving face." If someone is not having a good day, staff can call on him or her but should move on to the next *person* if there is no response.

Sharing Mementos from the *Person's* Home

Centers can take advantage of the fact that their participants are still living at home, homes filled with mementos from the *person's* past (e.g., varsity jackets, military dog tags, photographs from trips, and more). At times, these cherished articles can be shared for everyone to enjoy. Such sharing can also involve the families in the activities of the center.

Individualizing Activities

The day center should be a place in which individual needs can always be met. Working with the Best Friends model, staff should try to recruit volunteers to be a participant's Best Friend for a half-day a week to engage the *person* in a special activity. The *person's* life story can suggest potential volunteers. Many clubs and organizations, for example, will "take care of their own." Perhaps a college track team can adopt a retired coach enrolled in the day program who likes to take vigorous hikes every day.

Introducing Intergenerational Activities

Many adult day centers form linkages with child care centers. Group activities, conducted maybe once or twice a week, can bring joy to children and adults. Children seem to exemplify the knack of being nonjudgmental; they accept participants' memory losses. Also, almost all adults enjoy teaching and showing children something new.

Learning New Things

In life, we are always experiencing new things and learning new information. Although it is true that people with Alzheimer's disease may not be able to learn and retain new things, they may still enjoy the *experience* of being given new information. Program directors are encouraged to include upbeat current events, poetry readings, or "show and tell" in the group setting. Whether retained or not, the activity of learning new things builds self-esteem and keeps staff and volunteers interested.

Weekly Program or Theme

Key elements of knack include being flexible and creative and making something out of nothing. These elements are demonstrated wonderfully when centers develop weekly activities around a theme. Some day center participants enjoy a daily or weekly "program" that is put together by staff and volunteers. Typical subjects include seasonal fruit, money, old toys, hats, graduation, bells, school, presidents, national parks, shoes, winter clothes, famous people, and famous places. Daily or weekly programs can also be designed around holidays, such as Christmas, Halloween, and even Groundhog Day.

What makes the Helping Hand day center program special is the length to which the volunteers and staff go to make the most out of any program idea. An idea for a weekly program is subjected to the following battery of questions:

- What is the history of this individual, place, or thing?
- Is there an aspect of the program that can stimulate the five senses?
- Are there trivia questions that can be written about the topic?
- Are there songs that can be listened to or sung that relate to the topic?
- Are there objects or props that can be used to stimulate discussion?

- Are there old sayings or clichés that relate to the topic?
- Can any word games or other games be built around the topic?

A typical program centered around a theme is outlined in Figure 2.

CHALLENGES TO PROGRAM PARTICIPATION

Family Reluctance to Use Adult Day Services

One paradox that has confounded many people studying long-term care services is this: Why are so few families using adult day services if they are offering such a needed and affordable service? Some of the reasons may be related to the relative newness of these programs. Many people still do not know what adult day center care is. People over age 60 rarely used child care; they may be unlikely to use adult day services. Many communities may have only one adult day center and it may not be geographically convenient. Transportation may not be available. Some communities have centers that are open only part of the day. If a working caregiver needs adult day center care and his or her local program is open only 3 days a week from 9:00 A.M. to 3:00 P.M., the service may not be helpful *whatever* the quality or cost.

Even when adult day services are open for extended hours and readily available, many families are reluctant to use this important service. Family members give several reasons, including the following, for their reluctance to bring their loved one to an adult day center:

- **Denial** Denial can be very strong. "We're doing just fine," is commonly heard from families when this statement may or may not be true. The immediate caregiver may not be willing to see the extent of the problems. Professionals should remember that in small doses, denial is a healthy emotion—it gives us the ability to keep going in the face of adversity. Many caregivers believe that they do not really need help or they deny that a problem even exists; therefore, they feel why use adult day services?

- **Concern about money** Every adult day center administrator can share a story about a family that is reluctant to pay a sliding fee daily rate of $15, but that eventually pays $3,000–$4,000 a month to a nursing facility. Families sometimes delay or avoid using community services to save money, but it can be pointed out to them that it is a false economy "to save money for the nursing home." In fact, the use of services such as an adult day center may delay or prevent nursing facility placement altogether.

- **Caregiver reluctance to "let go"** Many caregivers spend so much time and effort providing care that it becomes hard to allow other people to lend a hand. They become accustomed to their burden and derive identity and meaning from martyrdom. These individuals may be guided by a sense of duty or they may simply be afraid that the center cannot handle their loved one.

- **The conviction that a day program will not work** Both authors have directed day center programs, and we have joked in the past that we wished we had a nickel for every family member who told us, "My dad will never come to the program. He was never a joiner. He'll never come or stay." Contrary to family expectations, we have almost always found that the *person* thrived in the program. Families should be reminded that dementia sometimes changes old attitudes. What a *person* would never do before, he or she now might do. For example, many families have noted that the *person's* past prejudices often dissolve and that they freely and comfortably interact with *people* from different class and ethnic backgrounds.

Encouraging the Use of Adult Day Services

Day center staff make a mistake when explaining their programs to prospective families by emphasizing the respite function. A typical "pitch" along this line would be to tell the caregiver, "You obviously need this service. Caregiving is very tiring, and you need a break." However well-meaning, in this case the day center director is being judgmental and may be pushing all sorts of emotional buttons of the family member, who may now feel even more guilty than before the meeting about giving up caregiving responsibilities.

The best approach for selling day center services is to stress the benefits to the *person*. A "pitch" to a family member could be made this way: "I think you're doing a terrific job, but our program can make an enormous difference to your family member through creative activities, loving care, and a chance to get out of the house to be with some new friends. Oh, by the way, it will give you as a caregiver a break."

The difference in the two approaches is clear. In the second approach, a caregiver is being given permission to use the service

Planning Ahead

1. Select a sample of several kinds of apples, such as red delicious, golden delicious, Granny Smith, and crab apple (if available).

2. Gather together as many props to use with apples as possible, such as
   - An apple basket
   - An apple peeler
   - A jar of apple butter and/or jelly
   - An old canning jar

3. Collect old sayings, songs, and poems about apples, such as
   - As easy as apple pie
   - An apple a day keeps the doctor away
   - Johnny Appleseed
   - Polishing the old apple
   - The Big Apple
   - "Don't Sit under the Apple Tree"
   - "In the Shade of the Old Apple Tree"

   Have props ready to use in the class session.

🍂 Class Session

1. Choose two apples from the collection and pass them around, giving time for everyone present to examine, smell, and comment.

   [sensory stimulation, socialization]

2. Wash apples and cut into bite-size pieces. Place apple pieces with a whole apple of the same type on a platter. Pass them around for tasting. As participants, staff, and volunteers taste, initiate conversation: "You are tasting the beautiful red delicious apple. Do you like the taste of this apple?"

   [enhanced self-esteem by giving an opinion]

3. After tasting two kinds of apples, ask everyone "Which do you like best?"

   [cognitive stimulation; opportunity to stimulate conversation]

4. After the taste test, pass around other kinds of apples to examine and enjoy and try to guess the name or how it could be cooked.

   [cognitive stimulation]

5. Bring out props to use with apples to reminisce. Ask questions to recall "old times":
   - "Did you have an apple tree on your farm?"
   - "Christine, I have eaten your apple pie. What a treat! Are you an apple pie baker, Edna?"
   - "How do you make apple butter?"
   - "What is a dried apple pie?"
   - "Did you ever eat too many little green apples?"

     [building self-esteem by contributing, being involved]

(continued)

Figure 2.   A typical program exemplifying creative activities in a day center setting.

6. Try to recall any old saying using the word "apple." Sing a song that has the word "apple" in it

   [*opportunity to recall familiar songs, quotes, and sayings*]

 Other Ideas

- Carve faces out of apples. After drying, they can be made into dolls (an Appalachian tradition).
- Talk about the custom of "bobbing for apples" at Halloween or about eating caramel apples.
- List some apple-producing states.
- Name all the products made from apples, such as apple cider, applesauce, fried apples, baked apples, apple butter, apple Jell-O, apple brown Betty.
- Make an easy apple dish such as baked apples.

Notes

Many ideas are presented here, but readers will think of others. Choose ideas that are compatible with the level of ability of your group and the amount of help available to you. This activity involves all people present equally. The most successful activities are fun for all.

Figure 2. (*continued*)

because it will be therapeutic for his or her loved one. Obviously, every family is somewhat different. Some families may be motivated strictly by respite concerns. However, it is critically important for day centers to be redefined as not just respite programs but as programs for the *person* with Alzheimer's disease as well.

Several other suggestions, as follows, can be made relating to the issue of encouraging families to use day services:

1. It is vital to stay in touch with families after they make initial contact or pay a first visit, perhaps inviting them back with their loved one for holiday dinners or special programs. Families sometimes take months or even a year to make a decision about adult day center care. A monthly call from the center director will usually be welcomed, and on one occasion the caregiver may say, "You know, I think it's time to try the program."

2. Support groups can help reinforce the benefits of adult day services. The family member considering adult day services can be encouraged to ask other families who are using the service for

their impressions. An enthusiastic family member who is satisfied with the service may spur the caregiver to try the program.

3. Finally, staff should bear in mind the complex dynamic at work in family decision making. When the Helping Hand program opened in 1984, volunteers would sing the praises of program participants when their families picked them up. "Your father did so well today. He did every activity, told a joke, cleaned up the kitchen, and had a smile for everyone." Contrary to expectations, caregivers seemed dumfounded and a little depressed by these cheery remarks. Staff learned that many people were quite sensitive to feelings that they were failing as caregivers—that we were doing a better job than they were. Thus day center staff should be positive but should not overdo it!

Individual Reluctance to Use Day Services

Once the center's staff have spoken with families about the service and convinced them to give it a try, the *person* must be convinced to come to the center and to stay. The ideas described in this section will lead to a good transition into adult day center care. Many families find that the decision to use adult day services is a good one. The families who have trouble convincing their loved ones to attend the day center may soon have trouble convincing them to leave!

Introducing the *Person* to Day Center Care

Families should be encouraged to come with the *person* to the center during the first or second visit. Families can review the knack of finesse in how they explain the service to the *person*, perhaps referring to it as "the class," "the job," or "the club." Finesse gives meaning and a sense of importance to the activity. Families may need to encourage the *person* or to make a statement in the morning such as, "Mom, we can't be late. Your class is starting soon." Families can tap into the *person's* sense of daily routine or daily obligation. For some *persons*, going to the day center is like going to work.

Another tactic is to have the family doctor write a "prescription" for day services. This way, the caregiver does not always have to be the "bad guy," telling the *person* what to do. The caregiver can now blame the doctor: "I'm sorry, dear. I know you don't want to go to that program today, but the doctor thinks you should give it a try." Also, this kind of statement does maintain caregiver integrity; almost all physicians dealing with Alzheimer's disease would support a family decision to use day services for the *person*.

Staff should encourage the family to remember the knack of good timing. It really is okay to tell the *person* he or she is going to the adult day center just moments before arrival!

Staff should also review the life story with the family to find specific "hooks" that may interest the *person* in the day program. A caregiver may then be able to say, "Mom, I am so excited for you! At your class today they are having a beautiful piano concert. I know how much you love the piano."

Helping the *Person* Become Acclimated

Staff should give some time and thought to the first impression the *person* will form when coming into the center. Body language is important. A big smile, open arms, and words of encouragement such as "It's great to see you, Dorothy. We've missed you" will put the *person* at ease.

Staff should use social graces to their advantage. Because we are all taught not to be rude, comments that evoke the *person's* sense of manners and good behavior can encourage the *person* to stay: "Mike, I'm so glad you're here today! I really need your help with a project. What would I do without you?" It is true that using social graces is manipulative, but many of us would have trouble not complying if a friend said this to us. We would probably stay and help him or her even if we did not want to.

Also, staff can use distraction to "cover" the caregiver's departure during the first days at the program. Often, family members find it hard to leave the center. The *person* may not want them to leave or may want to leave with them. A good distraction, such as asking the participant for help with a project, giving the participant a piece of coffee cake, or delivering a bear hug, can work wonders.

Involving the Family

The authors' experience from talking with day center directors around the United States is that day program staff generally enjoy excellent relationships with families. This success is partly the result of the fact that many families drop their loved ones off daily and pick them up. Thus the staff have continuing contact with family members.

The following are pointers for encouraging families to be more involved in the center:

1. **Be part of an effort to provide family education.** Day centers can sponsor lectures, support groups, workshops, and video screenings to help families better understand Alzheimer's disease and to help families improve caregiving skills.

2. **Involve families in any program to introduce the Best Friends approach at the center.** This easy-to-understand concept can build bridges and get families excited about volunteer recruitment and program development.

3. **Be a role model for families.** Many day center staff tell the authors that they often see families place their loved ones in long-term care facilities long before center staff think the time is right. Of course, centers are nonjudgmental and support family decisions, yet they can also be a perfect teaching/learning program or role model for families. Staff can teach families techniques and ideas that translate into the home setting, or let them spend time in the program if they are looking for new ideas. They will be doubly appreciative of the work center staff and volunteers do if they find that they are also learning to be better caregivers.

4. **Use the Best Friends model to discuss program philosophy and goals.** Every center should have a written philosophy that its staff can share with families that also explains intake and discharge decisions. An affirmative philosophy, such as the Best Friends model, will evoke positive responses from families and is easily understood.

5. **Consider developing a program to ease long-term facility placements.** Often, the day center staff become expert at understanding the participants in the program. The authors encourage centers to maintain a relationship with the family even after the *person* has become a resident in a facility. The benefits to having center staff sit in on the first care plan meeting at the facility and share insight into the *person's* strengths are many.

VOLUNTEER PROGRAMS

The authors suspect that many readers have turned directly to this section. In all areas of Alzheimer's care, programs are seeking new approaches to volunteer involvement. Volunteers bolster any program serving people with Alzheimer's disease by allowing for more individualized care. Volunteers also add quality enhancement to programs by bringing their own talents, skills, and interests to the program.

George Lubeley, a retired social services professional, described his satisfying work in the Helping Hand program: "Working one-to-one within a planned group activity, we were free to be ourselves and to relate to our 'friend' with spontaneity." He noted how rewarding it was to work with a participant "as a friend rather than a client."

This section examines volunteerism in day center settings, but is broadly applicable to many settings. Appendix A includes resources for further information about volunteer programs. The following are some ingredients of a successful volunteer program for centers and facilities embracing the Best Friends model:

1. **Give volunteers a meaningful, understandable role.** What is more simple, more understandable, and more meaningful than asking a potential volunteer to be a Best Friend to someone, or to take part in activities with a group of good friends? The authors encourage programs to recognize that volunteers want to do something valuable. They want to do more than just help out; they respond to and enjoy being a Best Friend to a participant.

2. **Develop a program that appeals to both participant and volunteer.** Activities must be appealing to volunteer and participant alike. Having activities that are too childlike or too boring will cause volunteers to lose interest quickly. The odds are strong that if the volunteers are happy, the participants are also happy.

3. **Give volunteers continual positive feedback.** A good program thanks volunteers often. It also constantly encourages volunteer input and listens to every individual's feelings and concerns. Incentives such as pins, mugs, and T-shirts are really not necessary. Most volunteers are motivated primarily by the value of the experience.

4. **Look to former caregivers to be volunteers.** After their loved one dies, some caregivers want to use what they learned in the program to help others. Sometimes caregivers whose loved ones have been placed in a long term care facility will help. This willingness may seem surprising, but readers should remember that these family members are skilled and at one time provided 24-hour care. Helping a few hours a week in a positive, upbeat, life-affirming program is a pleasure for many former caregivers.

5. **Build a family of volunteers.** Volunteers can become a close-knit group of friends. They gain satisfaction from the work they do, but they also build a sense of involvement and community by getting to know each other. The authors encourage centers to hold monthly luncheons or provide coffee and doughnuts weekly for the volunteers, and think of other events at which volunteers can socialize with one another. Perhaps staff and board members of day centers can all pitch in for one lunch hour a month so that the volunteers can all have lunch together in an adjoining room away from the program.

6. **Establish clear expectations.** When staff share expectations with volunteers, and clear job descriptions are provided, volunteers can be very reliable. It is advisable to develop a handbook for the volunteers that outlines program expectations. A monthly or quarterly newsletter, even one printed on the front and back of a piece of typing paper, goes a long way toward facilitating good communication and reinforcing program policies.

7. **Involve volunteers in all aspects of the program.** Volunteers can add much to the development and execution of activities, program committees, boards, and even fund-raising. Volunteers also model good care for students, families, and others visiting the day center. They bring a great deal of experience and talent to any program. (Appendix A lists resources for further information about volunteer programs.)

CONCLUSION: A NOTE TO FAMILIES

It is important to think about the impact of adult day center care on the *person*. Even if family members are providing exceptional care and believe they do not need respite, an adult day center environment can do things for the *person* that are not possible at home. Simply put, adult day services may be the best thing that can be done for *individuals* with Alzheimer's disease because the services force them to participate in society, engage them in activities and conversation, evoke old social graces, and stimulate them physically and cognitively.

Another reason exists to try adult day center services. As hard as it may be to consider the future, caregivers should remember the knack of planning ahead. It is possible that the *person* they care about will someday have to enter a nursing facility. *Persons* who have taken part in adult day services often make a better transition into long-term residential care. They have become accustomed to being away from the house and interacting in a group setting.

Finally, what is the risk in trying day center care? It simply involves trying a program several times and gauging what happens. If the program does not work, caregivers should mark their calendars 3 months ahead and try it again. Nothing ventured, nothing gained!

12

The Best Friends Approach in Long-Term Care Facilities

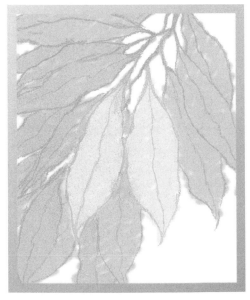

One of the authors' favorite stories concerning Alzheimer's disease comes from a caregiver support group meeting at which a family member ruefully cited the words of her doctor concerning long-term care placement: "It's time to put your husband in a nursing home. Your problems will be over then." That remark drew laughter and groans from the group.

Group members whose loved ones were already living in a facility had plenty of problems, including the following:

- Guilt about their decision
- Fear that their loved one will not be happy, will get hurt, will wander off, or otherwise will not make a successful transition into the facility
- Uncertainty about how to speak up when problems occur
- Fear that if the placement does not work out, the *person* may have to return home or move to a less desirable, or more distant, facility

- Uncertainty over how to get on with the rest of their lives

In addition, long-term care facilities, even those striving hard to deliver excellent care, face many challenges to providing good care for the resident with Alzheimer's disease, including the following:

- Lack of tools or easy-to-use concepts for working with residents with dementia
- Conflict with families
- Training and retaining good staff
- Overregulation, or regulations that may not be "dementia friendly," such as the conflict between fire codes and the desire to have secure doors and fencing
- Fear of litigation
- Lack of time to get everything done
- Maintaining morale

This chapter begins with a summary of how the Best Friends model can be applied to residential care settings, including staff training and development, activities, and family relations. It also includes a brief discussion of special care programs, a fairly new development that has both promises and pitfalls. This chapter is written for staff working in long-term residential care. However, families or others considering placement or who have placed loved ones in a facility will also find much information in this chapter helpful. It ends with a few special notes written for family members.

A note about terminology: The words describing long-term care facilities tend to vary by state or by region. In this chapter, the authors use the word "facility" to describe any supervised residential setting for the *person* with Alzheimer's disease. Most typically this term will encompass nursing facilities, which offer services including medical and rehabilitative care, and board and care homes, which offer supervised care and can be either small "mom-and-pop" operations or much larger homes.

THE BEST FRIENDS MODEL IN FACILITIES

Facilities are encouraged to adopt the Best Friends philosophy of care as a way of introducing a positive, life-affirming model of care that will improve staff morale and family satisfaction, make caregiving easier, and improve the quality of life for facility residents. The model is also a workable one for administrators concerned about staff productivity and costs.

The Best Friends model as applied to long-term care facilities provides the following suggestions for directors:

1. Recruit staff who have the potential to develop knack. All other skills can follow, particularly because facilities should have existing training programs.

2. Train *all* staff in the basics of Alzheimer's disease and teach them to understand the experience of Alzheimer's disease. This can be accomplished through lectures, talks with family members, books, articles, videos, and role-plays. Remember the knack of being well-informed.

3. Ask all staff to embrace the Alzheimer's Disease Bill of Rights (Chapter 4) and post the Bill of Rights in conspicuous places for families, residents, and staff. Adopt it as a voluntary statement of facility goals.

4. Ask all staff to think about their close friends and the qualities that make these friendships good. Discuss how facility staff can recast their working relationships with residents. Remember that the model does not call for staff to become actual friends, but rather to treat all residents as they would a "best friend."

5. Ensure that the care plan emphasizes the *person's* remaining strengths and abilities and that the assessment is looked at as a document that will change over time as Alzheimer's disease progresses.

6. Provide *all* staff with access to the life stories of residents with dementia. Develop incentives for staff to learn them and encourage staff to use the life stories in all aspects of daily care. This knowledge can pay big dividends with families because they are always impressed when staff are well-informed about their loved ones.

7. Explain to staff what knack means. Brainstorm about instances in which staff have shown knack.

8. Utilize the activity ideas described in this chapter to revamp the facility's approach to this important subject matter. Emphasize

to staff that every interaction is an activity and that it need only take a few seconds to make a big difference for the resident with dementia.

Every facility is bound to have differing strengths and weaknesses and differing concerns. The authors encourage facility administrators, nurses, activity staff, and others to examine the Best Friends model and consider how it can fit into the facility. The model lends itself to facility campaigns and contests, staff development, and all aspects of resident care. The ultimate benefit of the model is to change facility staff from being task oriented to being people oriented.

STAFF TRAINING AND DEVELOPMENT

To achieve high-quality Alzheimer's care, every facility should make staff training a priority. Fortunately, the Best Friends model has much to offer in this area. The model is woven into all aspects of training and includes the following benefits:

- **Simplicity.** The concept of treating people with Alzheimer's disease as friends is a simple concept, one that every staff member can learn and put into his or her own words and thoughts.

- **Multiculturalism.** Although many facilities employ staff who represent a true melting pot of ethnic backgrounds, the concepts in this model are universal. Although traditions vary somewhat, every culture understands friendship.

- **Rewards.** Facilities can include the Best Friends model in their incentive programs, perhaps awarding a monthly prize for the staff member who has demonstrated unusual knack.

- **Friendly competition.** In Alzheimer's care, it is critical for staff to know about the background of each resident. Facilities can create friendly competitions, even games, to encourage staff to learn resident biographies. For example, a nursing assistant who can name three facts about a particular resident on the spot can be given an award by the director of nursing.

- **Role-plays.** The best way to train staff using the Best Friends model is through active role-playing. For example, by asking staff to imagine what it would be like to travel to a foreign country where no one speaks their language, the training facilitator can initiate a discussion that will reveal the difficulties that can occur. Also, asking staff what activities they value and how they would feel if they had to give them up can create further empathy. Finally, examples of knack and no knack are often fun to act out, and they make the point very well about the importance of good care. Some further ideas for role-plays can be found on page 187.

ACTIVITIES

Facility staff have told the authors that activities is an area in which great improvements have been made, but it is also an area in which many challenges remain. Some of the challenges that come with Alzheimer's care are keeping group activities going when individual skills and interests vary, motivating volunteers to stay involved, and striving for new activity ideas.

Some principles of the Best Friends model of activities in facilities include the following:

1. **The definition of an activity is broadened considerably.** In the Best Friends model, in which one thinks about the *person* as a friend, staff should work to build pleasurable interactions into every activity. Thus, bathing a resident can also be a time for a funny story. Getting someone up in the morning can begin with a friendly smile, a compliment, and a hug.

2. **Everyone is an activities staff member.** Although facilities tend to have specialized activities staff, all staff should take the initiative to engage residents in activities.

3. **Activities should be individualized whenever possible.** The life story can provide many clues about the *person's* past interests, which can be tied into activities. If staff know that one resident was a champion bowler, they can always ask him or her about past wins, ask for advice about the game, or perhaps even set up a game of bowling outdoors.

4. **Friendly competition is encouraged.** All of us have a competitive nature, some of us more than others. In good Alzheimer's care, friendly competition can be fun. For example, the above-mentioned outdoor bowling game can be set up as a group activity with one big winner. However, staff should be certain everyone gets a consolation prize!

5. **Volunteers should be encouraged to be a Best Friend to a resident.** Volunteers often complain that they are not given meaningful work to do. In nursing facilities, volunteers often work in group settings. Facilities should also recruit volunteers to provide extra attention to residents with dementia who will benefit from one-on-one activities. As noted in Chapter 6, the *person's* life story can provide valuable clues to volunteer recruitment. A facility with a volunteer program might ask a labor union to "adopt" a retired member living in the facility and to participate in its volunteer program.

6. **Group activities should evoke feelings of camaraderie.** Group activities can engender a sense of togetherness and community. One of two formations is best—chairs in a circle or chairs around a table. Rather than strictly playing games or doing activities, facility staff should look at the description of a comprehensive activities program described in Chapter 11.

7. **Outside speakers, musicians, or groups should have an understanding of Alzheimer's disease.** Often, outside musicians, singers, artists, or other groups will come to facilities for performances, and these activities can be very successful. To maximize the potential for success, the outside individual or group will need to learn a few pointers about Alzheimer's disease. For example, the residents may enjoy a sing-along led by an outside group, but not if the group goes too fast. The group should be aware that people with memory loss often enjoy hearing a song or chorus repeated more than once.

8. **Even short, simple activities (mini-activities) are very meaningful.** Facility administrators are very concerned with productivity and getting the job done, yet some activities can be done in seconds and provide meaningful stimulation (see "30 Activities that Can Be Done in 30 Seconds or Less," pp. 188–189). Imagine if every staff member engaged 10 residents a day in one of these activities. The cumulative time spent would be less than 5 minutes per employee per day, but across the facility it would add up to a larger investment in needed socialization and interaction.

9. **Mini-activities can engage the *person's* attention and cooperation.** Equally important is that mini-activities tend to be icebreakers for nursing assistants who may then have to perform

difficult physical care tasks. Staff who are well-trained in the Best Friends model, who empathize with the *person* and understand the experience of Alzheimer's disease, are better able to perform their tasks with skill and finesse. They will get the job done better and more quickly with the cooperation of the *person*.

10. **Extended activities are an investment.** Although meaningful activities can be done quickly, spending more time on a task can be an investment that will pay off in fewer problem behaviors. Thus, if a nursing assistant is expected to give a complete bath in 15 minutes, an administrator may rethink the task and redefine it as an activity. If it now takes 20 minutes and the nursing assistant has been able to reminisce, tell a funny story, give a foot massage or back rub, and make a connection, the extra 5 minutes might make the bath go more smoothly, be a morale booster for the nursing assistant, and raise the self-esteem of the resident.

Activities in residential care facilities should be based on residents' strengths and have a positive purpose. Facilities should utilize the Best Friends model to conduct a thorough review of program activities. State review boards examine programs to ascertain whether they meet residents' psychosocial and emotional needs under federal requirements mandated in the Omnibus Budget Reconciliation Act (OBRA) of 1987 and 1990. Best Friends activities do this in many ways and can be charted as providing the following:

- Sensory stimulation
- Cognitive stimulation
- Creative expression
- Physical exercise
- Group cooperation, interactions, conversation, and cohesiveness
- Opportunities for socialization
- Opportunities for reminiscing, life reviews, and memories
- Ways to use old skills
- Ways to build self-esteem
- Ways to build relationships within the facility
- Positive ways to express emotions

- Support for a resident's wishes to maintain autonomy and independence

FAMILY RELATIONSHIPS

Facilities have a vital concern in addition to their residents: Family caregivers are also a critical part of the workings of any facility. Many family members provide informal care, without which a facility could not meet the needs of all residents. Families are also a rich source of activity ideas and feedback on program successes and failures. The Best Friends model can build bridges between facility staff and the family in the following ways:

- **Families can be involved in any program to introduce the Best Friends approach at the facility.** Families respond when they perceive that facilities are making positive changes. When facilities share with families their training or program goals, they will likely gain family support, which will provide staff with positive feedback and encourage families to participate in activity planning and volunteer recruitment.

- **The Best Friends model can be used to discuss program philosophy and goals.** The Best Friends model provides a good jumping-off point for administrative staff to educate families about what the facility can and cannot accomplish. When a facility can present a comprehensive and understandable philosophy and plan such as the Best Friends model, this provides a good framework for sharing concerns. Families want to know that facilities have a philosophy or vision, that the facility will not give up easily, and that the volunteers and staff are being well-trained.

SPECIAL CARE PROGRAMS

Many institutions around the United States are devoting energy to developing stand-alone Alzheimer's care facilities, or incorporating special care programs within existing facilities. Appendix A includes resources for individuals wanting to know more about special care. The authors also recommend that facilities be familiar with the national Alzheimer's Association *Guidelines for Dignity*, a publication about setting goals for special care (see Appendix A). In addition, the pointers listed on page 190 are provided.

Role-Play Ideas for Staff Training

Helping the *person* who keeps repeating the same question

Helping the *person* who is always busy arranging and rearranging chairs in the front lobby

Greeting the *person* using knack and then no knack

Redirecting the nursing assistant who always shares sad, depressing, or ominous stories

Talking with the *person* who is having a "down in the dumps" day

Dealing with the nursing assistant who is condescending to residents

Helping the *person* who is waiting in the hallway for something to happen

Making introductions in a group setting

Showing a nursing assistant who is task oriented instead of *person* oriented

Doing some 30-second activities (e.g., shaking hands, massaging shoulders, showing a family picture)

Asking opinions, giving compliments, and giving congratulations

Talking with a family member who is always critical of the care being provided by staff

Dealing with the activity volunteer who is not flexible

Praising the staff member who knows a *person's* life story very well

Encouraging the staff member who does not know anything about the *person*

Dealing with the nursing assistant who wears earphones while giving the *person* a bath

Talking about a *person* in his or her presence with another staff member

Trying to win an argument with a resident with Alzheimer's disease

The Best Friends Approach to Alzheimer's Care, by Virginia Bell and David Troxel.
Copyright © 1997, by Health Professions Press, Inc., Baltimore.

30 Activities that Can Be Done in 30 Seconds or Less

Greeting the *person* by name

Making eye contact and smiling

Shaking hands

Asking someone to "show me" an object

Teasing: "Mr. Smith, I just saw you eat dessert first!"

Telling someone he or she is loved

Giving a sustained bear hug

Giving a compliment: "Wow! You're looking pretty spiffy today, Margie."

Asking an open-ended question: "How are you feeling today, Mike?"

Asking an opinion: "What do you think of my new necktie? Does it match my shirt?"

Playing a quick game of catch

Noticing an unusual bird out the window

Evoking a memory from the life story of the *person:* "Tell me more about that grandfather of yours who was a country doctor. Did he really make house calls?"

Giving a hand massage

Sharing a new hand lotion and talking about its pleasing scent

(continued)

Blowing bubbles

Slipping a little treat to someone (being certain it's dietetically okay)

Sharing a magic trick

Showing off family photos of a new grandchild

Blowing up a balloon and batting it around

Looking at a flower arrangement and comparing colors, textures, and scents

Asking for advice on a recipe

Telling a funny story or joke

Doing a quick dance to some fun music playing in the background

Noticing vivid colors in an unusual dress or shirt

Asking for help with a chore, such as folding a towel, helping make a bed, or squirting some wax onto a piece of furniture about to be polished

Trying on a hat or hats

Trying on a new shade of lipstick

Clowning around for a moment, making funny faces, or throwing your hands in the air and spinning around once or twice in a silly dance

Stepping outdoors for some fresh air

1. **Special care programs should have a written philosophy of care.** Administrators of special care programs should be able to describe what their care goals are to potential residents and families. They should be able to explain why they are special.

2. **Special care may not be special.** Most states do not have regulations governing what special care is; thus, a facility may claim to provide special care but not be delivering it. Family caregivers should be cautious.

3. **Special care programs should have more intensive staffing ratios.** Because Alzheimer's care is people oriented, a special care program should have a much higher staff–resident ratio.

4. **Special care programs should have sophisticated care planning.** Special care programs should place extra emphasis on care planning that is strength-based, involving an interdisciplinary team to set appropriate goals and monitor residents' progress.

5. **Special care programs should emphasize staff training.** Special care programs should offer intensive and extensive training to their staff members. Caregivers should be able to expect staff to understand the fundamentals of Alzheimer's disease and certainly all of the basics listed in Chapter 2.

6. **Special care programs should have a dementia-friendly physical environment.** The best special care units have architectural design elements that are dementia friendly. These elements might include wandering paths, secure perimeters, good lighting, and soothing colors. It is important to note that the best architectural design will fail if staff do not have knack; conversely, a good program could be held in a barn with the right staff.

Fortunately, more is being learned about special care programs, and it is the authors' hope that the lessons learned from these programs will spill over into all facilities for older adults. Too many of us have had the experience of walking into a facility and observing many residents sitting alone, seemingly starved for attention and human contact. This should never happen in special care programs, and it is our greatest hope that the lessons learned from special care will have positive benefits for all residents. After all, we want Alzheimer's care to be special everywhere.

CONCLUSION: NOTES FOR FAMILIES

The most important message that the authors give caregivers facing the decision of residential placement is that it is *their* decision. Doctors, other family members, friends, even neighbors will say things such as "You should place him when he no longer knows you." "You should place her when she becomes incontinent." "You should place him when he doesn't sleep through the night." "You have no choice. You must place her now." The authors resist these blanket statements for several reasons.

First, every situation is different. Family members have differing skill levels, coping mechanisms, values, personalities, and resources that may play a large role in making a decision to keep someone at home or make a placement. A good example was a caregiver we knew who masterfully tackled the toughest aspects of care for her husband. She handled many difficult personal care chores, dressed and bathed him, took him to the day center, and designed activities for him. Her "breaking point" came when he began to have trouble climbing the stairs to their second floor bedroom. The doctor suggested putting a hospital bed downstairs in the formal dining room. She indicated that was the one thing she could *never* do, and that if her cherished formal dining room (symbolic of the last remaining structure in her life) were disturbed, she would then make a placement. This is an unusual example, but it does show that the decision to make a placement is based on many, sometimes surprising, variables. There is no simple formula.

Second, we believe strongly that caregivers have the right to make their own decisions, even if they are not always good decisions. Finally, when a caregiver is coerced to make a placement, it can often have unintended and unpleasant consequences. We know of one family in which the adult children compelled their father to place their mother. The *father's* health actually declined significantly over the anxiety and depression he felt about the placement; he also had several automobile accidents making his daily 20-mile round trip to the nursing facility. Were *his* problems over with the placement? In this case, the family ended up with two sick members.

Several factors are important for families to consider when deciding on long-term care placement:

1. **Rethink past promises.** The promise to "always keep Mother at

home" might have been made with the best intentions and hopes, but inherent in that commitment is the idea that the family will do what is *best* for Mother. It may be a promise that should be broken, because keeping Mother at home may not be best for her.

2. **Consider benefits of placement to the *person*.** Caregivers should not dwell only on the negatives surrounding placement; they should also think about the aspects of a facility that might actually be good for the *person*. An institution can, for example, often provide better physical care, such as more frequent bathing; provide more activities and socialization; offer a more regular routine; and sometimes offer a more nutritious menu.

3. **Take advantage of local resources.** Caregivers can talk with representatives of the local Alzheimer's Association about facilities that offer good Alzheimer's care. Also, they can consult with their state Long-Term Care Ombudsman, an individual whose position is mandated by a federal program and who advocates for people in long-term care facilities. The Ombudsman's office maintains reports on recent licensing inspections of local facilities and can also provide information about the placement process. Other good resources for placement ideas and help would be the Area Agency on Aging or, in some communities, private geriatric care managers who will help for an hourly fee.

4. **Identify potential facilities early.** Families often wait until a crisis hits to start looking for the right facility. Because many facilities have waiting lists, it is very important to visit facilities ahead of time, make lists of possible placements, and talk to the intake staff to be placed on appropriate waiting lists. One can always say no if notified of an opening.

5. **Recognize that caregiving does not stop with placement.** Many caregivers are consumed with the thought that placement represents a personal failure. A nursing facility placement does not end family care, it merely changes it, sometimes for the better. In many cases, caregivers who have been exhausted by physical care can now spend more high-quality time with their loved ones doing activities, taking walks, talking, reminiscing, or enjoying a meal together.

Caregivers must remember that placement is always their decision. They do have choices.

IV

The Best
Friends Model—
A New Day

*Noting the importance of being
one's own Best Friend, committing
to high-quality care, and looking
ahead to life after Alzheimer's
disease*

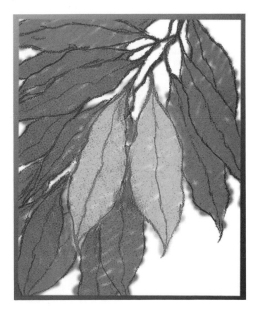

13

Being One's Own Best Friend

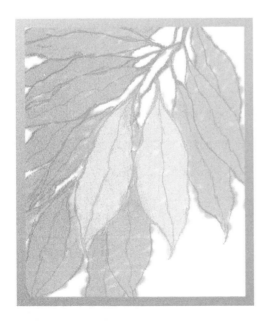

When traveling on commercial airlines, passengers are told that if air pressure is lost within the cabin, "Oxygen masks will lower . . . put your own oxygen mask on *first*, *then* put on your child's." The point the flight attendant is making is that if one does not take care of oneself first, he or she may not be in any position to help his or her dependent(s).

This image is a striking one for Alzheimer's care, because the caregiver's journey is a long one. We need to give ourselves *oxygen* first, to be strong and to survive in order to care for our loved ones. Alzheimer's disease is one of the most frightening and difficult of all diseases to cope with. There is no doubt that many individuals with Alzheimer's disease experience very difficult times; their families sometimes fare worse.

An important question the authors ask readers to consider is: What do we do in life when bad things happen to us? When adversity strikes—perhaps a financial reversal, the death of a loved one, or a job dismissal—some of us are consumed by anger, disappointment, or grief. Yet others have a way of working through the pain and coming out on the other side, sometimes much stronger. Growth, after all, usually comes from meeting and overcoming challenges.

The authors ask family caregivers reading this book to consider where they want to be in life 1 year, 3 years, or 10 years from now. The Best Friends model is a life raft being thrown to them, a chance to work hard to redirect disappointment, anger, or pain and instead find moments of joy in day-to-day life with their loved ones. We ask readers to be open to change. The Best Friends model cannot take away the diagnosis of Alzheimer's disease, but it can improve quality of life for caregivers and their loved ones. The Best Friends model encourages family caregivers to take care of themselves physically and emotionally, to maintain good-quality family relationships, and to work through the anger and pain that Alzheimer's disease can engender.

Professional caregivers should ask themselves if they are satisfied with their day-to-day working lives. Do they take joy in their work? The Best Friends model can help them gain more satisfaction from their work with individuals with dementia, improve their programs, and build their morale and the morale of facility staff as well. The Best Friends model encourages professional caregivers to embrace the Alzheimer's Disease Bill of Rights (see Chapter 4) and to take care of themselves first so that they can provide good-quality care to people with Alzheimer's disease.

The authors encourage *persons* with emerging Alzheimer's disease reading this book to adopt the philosophy of Rebecca Riley—to live one day at a time; to teach others, like Beverly Wheeler; to maintain faith in a higher power, like Dicy Jenkins; to maintain a sense of humor, like Joe Blackhurst; to expose oneself to learning, like Helen King; and to maintain a determined spirit, like Mary Katherine Davis. One should use one's strengths as long as possible and surround oneself with Best Friends.

One of the important benefits of the Best Friends model is that it provides protection to the caregiver. When professional and family caregivers can integrate elements of good friendship into skilled care, be flexible, have a sense of humor, and understand that it is important to relate to the *person,* not just the disease, caregiving becomes easier and more rewarding. The Best Friends model is life affirming and can prevent feelings of hopelessness. Satisfaction and pride can come from giving good care, being supportive, being there for the *person* with Alzheimer's disease.

This chapter offers ideas that can help caregivers take better care of themselves. The authors refuse to list a series of "musts." Just as we have argued that every *person* with Alzheimer's disease is different, it can be argued that every *caregiver's* situation is different. Each caregiver alone should decide which idea is applicable to his or her situation.

This chapter will not repeat all the major suggestions from the previous 12 chapters. The authors hope caregivers will remember to learn as much as they can about Alzheimer's disease, empathize with the *person*, be an advocate for the Alzheimer's Disease Bill of Rights, make a careful assessment, develop a comprehensive life story, and work on developing the knack of care. We also hope caregivers will not fall into the trap of waiting too long to use (or not use at all) valuable services that can enrich the life of the *person* with the disease and give the caregiver respite.

Readers will find material on being one's own best friend in almost every chapter of this book. However, this chapter gives some specific strategies on this topic that build on previously covered material. This chapter primarily addresses family caregivers in the list of ideas on being one's own best friend; however, almost all of the strategies can be adopted by professional caregivers as well.

How to Be One's Own Best Friend

Maintain a Sense of Humor

The art of providing good care involves maintaining a sense of humor and striving to "lighten up" about life's challenges. Watching a classic comedy movie or program on television, sharing a funny story at a support group meeting, or simply laughing with the *person* can help inoculate one against the stress and strain of caregiving.

Seek Out Someone to Confide In

A trusted friend or counselor can make all the difference to a family caregiver. He or she needs someone to talk things over with, someone who will be nonjudgmental, respect confidentiality, and be understanding of one's needs. Families who in the past would never have considered counseling should throw out these attitudes. A good counselor can help in many ways.

Set Realistic Expectations

Because we care about our loved ones, we can very easily lose sight of how much giving of ourselves is realistic and healthy. A caregiver should survey him- or herself using the following questions: What is the state of my health? How much of the physical care can I reasonably provide, if any? How much time can I spend on caregiving (away from employment or other family obligations)? What kind of family support do I get, if any? How much money can I spend on caring for my loved one without jeopardizing my family's financial well-being?

Practice Assertiveness

Often, it is hard to express one's feelings and needs to others. When stress or fatigue increase, caregivers may become even less communicative. Caregivers should practice assertiveness, and not be afraid to speak up to family members and friends about their feelings and needs. It is okay to admit that one is not okay.

Develop Strategies for Handling Unhelpful Advice

Advice from a trusted friend or professional can be helpful, but caregivers sometimes find themselves deluged with unsolicited suggestions. Friends and family mean well, but their unwanted suggestions or comments such as "Put him in a nursing home" or "She doesn't seem that bad to me" can create more stress. Helpful advice is a gift, but if the advice is not helpful, develop a few stock responses such as "Thanks for your input," or "Thanks for your concern."

Keep Up Contact with the Outside World

Caregivers who devote all their energy toward their loved one can inadvertently shut out friends and family. Often, caregivers must cut back on commitments and social activities, but balance is important. They should try to make at least one call each week to a friend that they have been too busy to see or talk to. Also, many caregivers find new friends through support groups, introductions to families at day centers, or other programs that help families cope with Alzheimer's disease.

Modify or Change the Living Environment

Usually, it is not prudent for caregivers to move a household immediately after receiving a diagnosis of Alzheimer's disease. There is ample time to make decisions and carry them out. Caregivers should instead consider whether their home is "dementia friendly"—Is it conveniently located to services? Is it close to people who can help? Is the home safe? Is it hard to maintain? Individuals or families should weigh carefully a decision to leave a longtime hometown just to be closer to one or two family members. It can be hard to develop a new network of friends in a new location. Alternative housing such as a retirement community or assisted living should be considered.

Fulfill Creative Impulses

Many caregivers find that creative expression can be a positive way to cope with Alzheimer's disease. Caregivers have written poems, plays, novels, even an opera; produced films; and painted about their experiences. Creative work can help caregivers channel their anger and despair into more positive outlets.

Listen to One's Body

People providing care to individuals with Alzheimer's disease are at greater risk for premature disability and death than are noncaregivers of the same age. This risk is the result of numerous factors, notably the stress that comes from the tasks of caregiving. Caregivers are encouraged to eat properly, exercise, and pamper themselves. Some family caregivers have received benefits from getting regular massages, meditating, getting makeovers, and other rewards.

Be Good to Oneself

Caregivers should zealously carve out time for themselves and try to maintain special activities, hobbies, friends, or other activities that give pleasure. Caregivers should also give themselves presents, such as a new big-screen television set; an afternoon spent fishing; or fresh flowers from the local farmers' market, whenever possible.

Plan Ahead

Because the progression of Alzheimer's disease is often slow, families usually have time to plan ahead. For example, some caregivers never consider the possibility that they might predecease the *person*. Without a workable plan for this circumstance, a family's financial affairs and care plan for the *person* can be disrupted.

Forgive Others and Oneself

Alzheimer's disease finds people at their best and at their worst. When their friends or family say or do the wrong thing, caregivers can find it valuable to look at the underlying motive. That motive may be love and concern, even if what is said or done is not helpful. It is also true that the best caregivers are often hardest on themselves. Caregivers should give themselves permission to make mistakes; to have bad days; and to think angry, even shameful thoughts. Even the closest friends have their ups and downs.

Keep a Diary or Notes of Caregiving Experiences

Many family caregivers find that keeping a diary or notes about the experience of giving care can be helpful. It can help caregivers solve problems. A diary can provide a safe place to write about stresses, strains, and feelings—good and bad—and to "vent," to say the things the caregiver wants to but cannot say in public.

At the end of this chapter are excepts from the diary and a series of Christmas card letters written by Jo Riley, husband of and caregiver to Rebecca Riley. Throughout this book, we learned about Rebecca Riley and her experiences coping with Alzheimer's disease. Jo turned to writing to record Rebecca's progress and his reactions to her illness.

HOW TO COPE WHEN
EVERYTHING IS GOING WRONG

Even people who practice the Best Friends model will find the challenges of caregiving overwhelming at times. Alzheimer's disease can provide tremendous challenges to the most skilled caregiver. For example, if the *person* has an undetected infection or is in pain, behaviors can throw the most well-planned activity into chaos. Sometimes caregivers get into such a slump (e.g., because of depression, fatigue, frail health) that they find it hard to take action. Their judgment can become clouded.

One of the most important ways to be one's own best friend is to take advantage of available respite care opportunities. The authors' first choice is always adult day center care, which we have described as a "treatment" for Alzheimer's disease. Day services also gives a valuable and important break to the caregiver. Respite opportunities can be informal as well, such as saying yes to a friend or family member who offers to come and help for an afternoon.

The following list of ideas of how to cope when everything seems to be going wrong have come from caregivers with whom the authors have worked. Some ideas are serious, others a little outrageous, but all have worked for some caregivers. These ideas are examples of "stress busters." They help us learn to be our own best friends. When everything is going wrong:

- Take a day off and do whatever you want.
- Wait until a train is passing; go outside and scream as loud as you can.
- Call a friend to come over to be with you.
- Read a joke book.
- Hug a friend.
- Call your minister/priest/rabbi to share your feelings.
- Buy a new outfit.
- Take a long walk in nature.
- Order a pizza and eat it all.
- Spend a weekend at a retreat center.
- Be humble enough to accept help and support.
- Have a good, therapeutic cry!

CONSIDER THE FUTURE

Earlier in this chapter, the authors asked readers to consider where they want to be in life 1 year, 3 years, or 10 years from now. Each of us should think about what relationships we want to have at that time with our family and friends. What do we want to be able to say about our time as caregivers?

The Best Friends model suggests that the caregiving experience is like one door closing and another opening. One caregiver jotted down the following words when thinking about his future: New friends and relationships, travel, new hobbies, laughter, tears, healing, and pride in a job well done.

Being one's own best friend maximizes quality of life during the sometimes arduous tasks of caregiving. Even more important, it positions one for a life after Alzheimer's disease.

DIARY ENTRIES

The following pages contain excerpts from Jo Riley's writings from the date of Rebecca's diagnosis in 1984 through 1995. The authors find his words valuable because they demonstrate that one can be a good and dedicated caregiver while being intentional about acting as one's own best friend. Except for minor editing for clarity, the words are Jo's.

July 30, 1984   A devastating day for the Rileys. We had an appointment with a neurologist in St. Louis. We had been to see him in June and had a CT scan and other tests made. Some of these were made in his office and others were made in Barnes Hospital. He did not have the results of the test for several weeks. We were going to Jamaica and we went with great expectation. When we went to see him on our return he just very quietly said that Rebecca had Alzheimer's disease. We were devastated! We knew something was wrong and we were hoping that it would be a brain tumor or something else.

When we learned of her diagnosis, I recalled that Rebecca began having trouble about a year and a half ago pronouncing some words. She was an excellent reader, fast reader, and a good reader. She stumbled over some of these words and I didn't think anything about it. I recall now that was the first sign of trouble.

We left Barnes Hospital and drove toward Centralia . . . and had lunch. It was a sober lunch and a very quiet one. We resolved that we were going to make the best of it and live one day at a time.

November 1984   We were in Jewish Hospital in St. Louis. Joy, our doctor daughter-in-law, said that there was an aging support group there. We inquired of it and had an interview with a nurse and a social worker. The interview lasted about an hour and toward the end of it I had to direct the nurse's and the social worker's attention to what was happening in the interview. They had not talked directly to Rebecca but had always asked me and directed the conversation toward me. This made Rebecca feel left out. When I called it to their attention, they were surprised and shocked. Their only explanation was that when they had dealt with families with Alzheimer's disease, they had only talked to the caregiver. Rebecca was the youngest person they had talked to that had been diagnosed. I think this is the first time that I had felt that social workers and nurses and doctors were thinking only of the families, they are not thinking of the patient.

We were trying to see if there was a support group. There was a support group for caregivers coping with Alzheimer's disease but none for the patient.

Spring 1985   We planned our move to retire in Kentucky. At this time I have been noticing that Rebecca was still having trouble in reading and that she was having some trouble in writing. She was constantly referring to the dictionary and having trouble finding words. Our children have been fully supportive and wanted us to come by and see them.

June 1985   We went to the lake. This is Crystal Lake in Northern Michigan. We had a summer that was filled with visits. Our families knew of her condition, but Rebecca was beginning to feel left out. I think she wanted to talk to them about it but they were afraid to. This is another example of the loneliness that crept into her.

January 1986   We went to Hopkinsville, Kentucky for an interim ministry. While we've been in Hopkinsville I've noticed some things. First she is more withdrawn. She has always been an outgoing person, speaking and teaching. I've noticed that she is kind of withdrawn, she's scared of people because she can't remember names. She's writing names down every place but has trouble remembering them. Her reading may be a little worse and her writing is good, legible, but she has a hard time getting out the words she wants.

We've not told anybody in Hopkinsville, but she has been accepted and loved. The trouble with cancer, Alzheimer's disease, and many other diseases is when people know it they immediately shy away from the person. Rebecca knows this as a nurse, she sees it now that she has Alzheimer's and it is a very depressing state. We as a people do not know how to treat people who are sick. They want to talk about it, but we are afraid to talk about it.

The dictionary is now her constant companion.

We need something for Rebecca. We feel that there is a need for a support group for the patient. There may not be enough people who develop Alzheimer's disease in time to be helped by this type of group.

Summer of 1986   We went to our cottage at Crystal Lake. We had all the family there and it was a good time. I noticed that it takes Rebecca longer to plan and execute the plan.

One thing that I have noticed is that Rebecca has talked more in the past year about getting a dog or pet. She has empathy for people and animals. She has always had it but she's commented about the butterflies, driving she doesn't want to kill one or an animal. She loves birds and loves to watch them. I've noticed that she wants me with her more than ever. I guess she wants reassurance.

October 1986   She is carrying on as usual. She's cooking, she's doing her needle-point, she's singing in a church choir and she is going with me whenever I go out of town. Sometimes I notice she doesn't want to talk and other times she enters into conversation.

We are getting ready to go back to Lexington and she is doing the packing. Of course there are some things she can't remember where she put them but we are living in a mess anyway.

She is carrying the checkbook and is doing a very good job writing a check. She said she is afraid of writing a check but so far she has been very accurate. I think in writing the check she gets confused on having to write out the words on the check. She gets stopped on the spelling of "hundred" or whatever the figure is. She wrote all our thank-you's and kept them up to date.

We have always made decisions together and we want to keep the "we" in our relationship.

We are planning to go to Australia in three months. We are looking forward to it.

She is taking exercise classes five days a week. The people here have been gracious and she has said several times she hates to leave. She says she is worried about me in Lexington because we do not have many friends there.

Thus far we know of no medicine, no treatment, or no cure. We're living one day at a time.

CHRISTMAS SALUTATIONS

1987   At Christmas, Joetta and Bill called us to say that they wanted to bring two friends with them. We said OK. It turned out to be two dogs; when they left, we were the proud owners of "Corky," a Chinese Shih'tzu. He thinks that he is a person and is always at our feet.

We are making Lexington our home base. Christmas is a time to visit with each other so we have tried to do it in this newsletter. We would like to welcome you to our home (be sure to call ahead of time).

Christmas is the spirit of love which God has gratefully given to each of us and we extend to you. At Christmas time, the angels sang of peace and goodwill which is translated, "love to you."

Rebecca and Jo

1988   Jo served as interim minister for two months at Woodmount Christian Church in Nashville. It was a great experience working with the staff in this large metropolitan church. The byproduct was visiting many historical sites around Nashville.

After three weeks home in Lexington we were off to the USSR for a pilgrimage to the Russian Orthodox Church which celebrated their 1000th year.

Rebecca had a big time in May when her family had a family reunion.

Christmas is the spirit of love which God has gratefully given to each of us and we extend to you our love.

Rebecca and Jo

1989   We got back home from Crystal Lake. Our summer was filled by drinking in beautiful sunsets, the blues of Crystal, the sand dune, the birds of the sky, and enjoying the many friends in Michigan.

In August we came home for a weekend and packed up for our big trip to Alaska. At Nome we felt the excitement of being in the "Gold Rush Capital" and hearing of the millions of dollars which was mined in the 1890 rush. Yes, we "panned" for gold and got two flakes!

We are enjoying our retirement with Corky, a little Shih'tzu, who requires a walk twice a day. May the love of Christmas be yours and warm your hearts and fill your life with Love.

Rebecca and Jo

1990   The most wonderful season of excitement is upon us. The Spirit of Christmas is found in carols of Joy, Peace, and Good News.

The big news of 1990 for the Rileys was our move. In February we decided to move to Richmond Place, an elder retirement apartment which advertises as a place for "gracious retirement living."

Rebecca went on all our trips this year and enjoyed them. As you know, Rebecca has Alzheimer's disease. She is very forgetful and it is hard to plan anything in the future. The move was frustrating and difficult for her because she thought that we were giving everything away. Now the move is over, she has settled down and is liking our living situation.

As Christmas comes, we rejoice in knowing that there is love all about us. That's what Christmas is all about. We pray that the Heart of Christmas will be in your home and your heart.

Rebecca and Jo

1991   Time is marching on and the calendar reveals it to us. In February we were invited back to Kokomo to help them celebrate their 140th anniversary. It is hard to believe we were there for their 100th birthday.

The last of May we arrived at Crystal Lake and found everything as peaceful as ever. We entertained 15 groups of people for dinner during the summer with Jo being the "chief cook and bottle washer." Rebecca tried swimming and sailing only once.

Rebecca has become a little more confused and depended upon me for everything. She went everywhere that I went but wanted to stay home most of the time. The children insisted that I investigate a health care facility. After long hours of anguished prayer, I selected one that had a personal care bed. On October 3rd, I made the hardest and saddest decision of my life—to take Rebecca to a health care center.

Within 3 days, the nurses said that Rebecca couldn't care for herself and that she would have to move to intermediate care. I go once or twice a day (except Sundays).

My life has changed for we did everything together. My ministry was always a co-ministry.

During the last week of October I went to the General Assembly of the Christian Church which met in Tulsa.

We wish for you a Merry Christmas and may the Spirit of the Christ child be in your heart.

Rebecca and Jo

1992 In a comparative religion course I am taking at UK, our textbook states the uniqueness of Christianity is that we are able to be a "real lover of humankind."

Since October 3, 1991 Rebecca has been in the Christian Health Center suffering from Alzheimer's. She initially lost some weight but has stabilized now.

Lucinda and Josh took the nice "old man" on a family hiking trip and camping trip in August to the Cascade Mountains of Washington state. We hiked every day.

Oh, by the way, Corky, our little dog was given to Joy's uncle in Anderson, Indiana. Now I am all alone.

In the spring and fall, I enrolled in a UK class which meets twice a week.

We hope for every one of you a Joyful and Peaceful Christmas.

Rebecca and Jo

1993 As understanding and love come down at this season, it has strengthened our family relationships and at Christmas time we pause to remember what has happened to the Riley family during 1993.

Our primary concern is Rebecca who remains at Christian Health Center with Alzheimer's disease. Her health is still good, but we do not take her out of the center often.

I go twice a day to feed her. While she is walking, she notices other patients in wheelchairs and tries talking to them. She doesn't recognize anyone but me and sometimes not even me.

During the year, I haven't allowed much grass to grow under my feet, attending elderhostels on Catalina Island, CA, and one at the Art Institute of Chicago.

I want all of us to feel the Spirit of Christmas and in our hearts to experience the Love, the Hope, and Faith of a Joyful Christmas.

Yours in Christmas love,
Rebecca and Jo

1994 Christmas is all about Good News and has Joy for its theme. Throughout the past year, we all have had our "ups and downs," but when we recall the message of Christmas, we can have truly a spirit of Hope.

My schedule has revolved around going to visit Rebecca. I go to feed her breakfast which means leaving the apartment around 6:50 am and return at 11 am for her lunch. She brightens up when she sees me but hasn't called my name for more than a year and a half. (I doubt she knows me but laughs and smiles as she recognizes me as a person who comes to see her.)

In March, I spent a week in Florida as a volunteer for Habitat for Humanity.

In May, a reporter from the Lexington newspaper interviewed several of us from Richmond Place who have bequeathed their brains at their death to Alzheimer's research. There was a large picture of me and two others in the magazine section. I said I wasn't quite yet ready to give up my brain!

May you find the spirit of Love and a feeling of Hope this Christmas.

Jo

1995 Love is what makes the world go round is a line of an old song. That's what Christmas is all about, Love, the glue that ties a family together, the bond between friends, the goodness that we express to others, the caring for others, and the spirit of friendship.

This has been a full year with many varied experiences. Rebecca is still living at Christian Health Center. She is slowing down and spends her time in a jerrie chair and uses her walker very little.

At the time of our 50th anniversary all of the children surprised us with a visit. On Saturday noon we decided to have a picnic in the park as it was a beautiful day. We took Rebecca out. We hope she enjoyed it.

That evening, they surprised me with a dinner with many close friends. The evening added to my special recollections of Rebecca.

Josh, our grandson, and I had a trip in October we will never forget. We traveled 1000 miles by van to Churchill, Canada, to see polar bears in migration. We saw six polar bears and two white foxes.

At this Christmas season, I wish for you all the Christmas Joy and Love.

Jo

Authors' Note (Summer 1996) Jo continues his twice-daily visits to Rebecca. He will work on a house for Habitat for Humanity this summer, and later in 1996 will attend two Elderhostel programs, one near the Chesapeake Bay in Maryland and the other in Spain. By connecting with life on his own, enjoying volunteer and educational experiences, Jo can continue to be Rebecca's Best Friend as well as his own Best Friend.

14

Light Out of Darkness

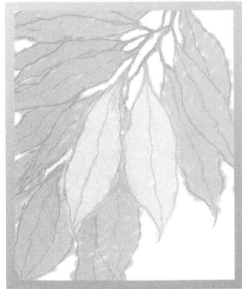

Hope is not pretending that troubles do not exist. It is the trust that they will not last forever, that hurt will be healed, and difficulties will be overcome. It is faith that a source of strength and renewal lies within us to lead us through the dark to the sunshine.

Anonymous

The authors urge family and professional caregivers to incorporate the Best Friends model into their everyday caregiving. If it is successfully learned, it can greatly improve quality of life for the *person*, the family, and the caregiver(s). Day centers and facilities will find that the model attracts tremendous family and staff support. Friendship is universally understood, and the ideas in this model are easy to learn and to put into practice.

We have too long dwelled on the darkness and despair that can be part of living with Alzheimer's disease. There is another face to Alzheimer's disease, with more and more families and professionals calling for a more positive approach to care and to caregiving. The Best Friends model makes this hopeful philosophy possible. For the families who may still doubt the power of this model, the authors offer this challenge: What is the risk of trying the Best Friends model?

The medical condition of the *person* with Alzheimer's disease cannot change, but the approach of professional and family caregivers can. If caregivers make the changes suggested by the Best Friends model, the authors believe that problem behaviors can be reduced and that a joyful, safe, secure, and rich life can be created for the *person*.

Chapter 1 describes many of the feelings common to people with Alzheimer's disease, including loss, isolation and loneliness, sadness, confusion, worry and anxiety, frustration, fear, paranoia, anger, and embarrassment. Most of us experience one or more of these feelings at times. People with Alzheimer's disease who are not receiving good care may be easily overwhelmed by negative emotions. The Best Friends model restores balance; the interventions used can convert negative feelings into more positive emotions.

As stated in Chapter 1, one of Rebecca Riley's greatest fears was that she would not be treated as a "real person" by others. Following are examples of how the Best Friends model reinforced positive emotions and helped Rebecca feel valued, part of her family, and connected to the world around her.

The Best Friends model can turn feelings of loss into feelings of fulfillment

- Rebecca gained a sense of worth from teaching a class for young adults at church for the first year after her diagnosis.
- Rebecca took pride in remembering lyrics when singing in the church choir.
- Rebecca maintained her family role as grandmother to her grandchildren.
- Rebecca felt rewarded when helping others, especially at the day center.

The Best Friends model can turn feelings of isolation and loneliness into feelings of connectedness

- Rebecca felt important and competent when Jo made her feel part of his ministry.

- Rebecca felt friendship and support from a couples group.

- Rebecca received unconditional love from her dog, Corky.

- Rebecca connected to the community by attending classes and concerts with Jo.

The Best Friends model can turn feelings of sadness into feelings of cheerfulness

- Rebecca could be a "free spirit," feeling few expectations of her at the Crystal Lake cabin.

- Rebecca reminisced gleefully when her younger sister recalled funny childhood stories.

- Rebecca smiled when friends talked with her about her nursing career and her family, discussing the children by name.

- Rebecca felt less depressed when friends stopped by for a visit in the secure environment of her home.

The Best Friends model can turn feelings of confusion into feelings of orientation

- Rebecca enjoyed skills such as swimming, hiking, and boating when surrounded by family and friends.

- Rebecca responded well when others slowed down in conversations.

- Rebecca appreciated when day center staff gave her cues to relive important life events.

- Rebecca felt the most oriented at Christian Health Center when surrounded by familiar family mementos.

The Best Friends model can turn feelings of worry and anxiety into feelings of contentment

- Rebecca found listening to music and playing still-familiar songs on the piano soothing.

- Rebecca marveled at the beautiful sunsets at Crystal Lake.

- Rebecca delighted in simple activities such as watching birds and butterflies.

- Rebecca felt comforted when being read to aloud.

The Best Friends model can turn feelings of frustration into feelings of serenity and peacefulness

- Rebecca loved the serenity at Crystal Lake.
- Rebecca felt joy when her children called or sent flowers for holidays or special occasions.
- Rebecca found long walks peaceful.
- Rebecca enjoyed working in the yard at a slow pace.

The Best Friends model can turn feelings of fear into feelings of security

- Rebecca felt safer when friends and families acknowledged her illness.
- Rebecca appreciated that she was never left alone in public.
- Rebecca felt reassured by friendly hugs.
- Rebecca loved feeling "protected" by her dog, Corky.

The Best Friends model can turn feelings of paranoia into feelings of trust

- Rebecca felt more involved in family finances when Jo let her sign the checks he filled out to pay bills.
- Rebecca liked that Jo used "we" instead of "I" when talking about their family.
- Rebecca appreciated making decisions, even simple ones, or being asked her opinion.
- Rebecca felt that friends were *their* friends, instead of *Jo's* friends, when Jo asked her to contribute to the annual Christmas letter.

The Best Friends model can turn feelings of anger into feelings of calm

- Rebecca released pent-up energy when walking the dog.
- Rebecca felt calm when volunteers at the day center respected her sense of pride, even in a matter as simple as hanging up her own coat.
- Rebecca found that vigorous exercise diffused anger.
- Rebecca felt distracted by the simple act of holding hands, cuddling, or being loved.

The Best Friends model can turn feelings of embarrassment into feelings of confidence

- Rebecca liked it when Jo would help her prepare a simple meal.
- Rebecca was helped by having people around her who understood Alzheimer's disease.
- Rebecca felt competent and useful when exposed to day center programs that matched her remaining skills.
- Rebecca felt more equal when Jo told a joke at his own expense.

The authors have referred to the Best Friends model as a road map of sorts, a way of getting from "here" to "there." In a sense, it is also a way of getting the *person* from "here" to "there." The model can help to shift negative behavior to positive behavior. Friendship applied to Alzheimer's care can be a powerful tool.

The authors wish every caregiver knack. Family and professional caregivers with knack are confident people who deliver confident care, prevent problems before they occur, and enjoy spending time with the *person*.

The Best Friends model was created primarily for family and professional caregivers coping with the effects of Alzheimer's disease, but there are lessons in it for everyone. There is great value in being totally present for another individual. There is great value in getting the most out of every moment, every day. There is great value in good communication. There is great value in honoring an individual's life story. There is great value in giving care to another.

Because any of us can be touched by Alzheimer's disease, can have bad things happen to us, our friends, or our families, the ultimate message the authors wish to convey is this: We should treat everyone important to us as we would our own Best Friend.

Appendixes

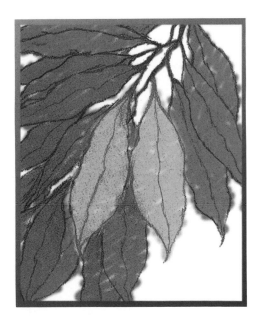

Appendix A: Resources for Families[1]

Alzheimer's Association
919 North Michigan Avenue
Suite 100
Chicago, Illinois 60611-1676
Phone (312) 335-8700
Phone (800) 272-3900

Alzheimer's Disease Education and Referral Center (ADEAR)
National Institute on Aging
Post Office Box 8250
Silver Spring, Maryland 20907-8250
Phone (800) 438-4380
Fax (301) 587-4352

American Art Therapy Association, Inc.
1212 Allanson Road
Mundelein, Illinois 60060
Phone (847) 949-6064

American Association of Homes and Services for the Aging
901 E Street, NW
Suite 500
Washington, DC 20004-2037
Phone (202) 508-9400
Fax (202) 783-2255

American Association for Music Therapy[2]
Post Office Box 80012
Valley Forge, Pennsylvania 19484
Phone (914) 944-9260

---

[1] This list of resources is accurate to the best of the authors' knowledge, and does not suggest any endorsement by the authors or the publisher.
[2] By 1998 the National Association for Music Therapy will unite with the American Association of Music Therapy to become the American Music Therapy Association.

American Association of Retired Persons (AARP)
601 E Street, NW
Washington, DC 20049
Phone (202) 434-2277

American Dance Therapy Association
2000 Century Plaza
Suite 108
Columbia, Maryland 21044
Phone (410) 997-4040

American Society on Aging (ASA)
833 Market Street
Suite 512
San Francisco, California 94103
Phone (415) 974-9600
Fax (415) 974-0300

Association for Volunteer Administration
Post Office Box 4584
Boulder, Colorado 80306
Phone (303) 541-0238

Brookdale National Group Respite Program
2320 Channing Way
Berkeley, California 94704
Phone (510) 540-6734
Fax (510) 540-6771

Children of Aging Parents (CAPS)
1609 Woodbourne Road
#302A
Levittown, Pennsylvania 19057
Phone (215) 945-6900

Gerontological Society of America (GSA)
1275 K Street, NW
Suite 350
Washington, DC 20005
Phone (202) 842-1275
Fax (202) 842-1150

National Association of Activity Professionals (NAAP)
1225 I Street, NW
Suite 300
Washington, DC 20005
Phone (202) 289-0722
Fax (202) 842-0621

National Association of Area Agencies on Aging
1112 Sixteenth Street, NW
Suite 100
Washington, DC 20036
Phone (202) 296-8130
Fax (202) 296-8134

National Association for Home Care
519 C Street, NE
Washington, DC 20002-5809
Phone (202) 547-7424

National Association for Music Therapy, Inc.[2]
8455 Colesville Road
Suite 930
Silver Spring, Maryland 20910
Phone (301) 589-3300

National Association of Professional Geriatric Care Managers
1604 North Country Club Road
Tucson, Arizona 85716
Phone (520) 881-8008
Fax (520) 325-7925

National Center on Elder Abuse
810 First Street, NE
Suite 500
Washington, DC 20002
Phone (202) 682-0100

National Council on the Aging
(National Adult Day Services Association)
409 Third Street, SW
Second Floor
Washington, DC 20024
Phone (202) 479-1200

National Institute on Aging (NIA)
Public Information Office
Building 31, Room 5C27
31 Center Drive
Bethesda, Maryland 20892
Phone (800) 222-2225
(publications on aging)

The Points of Life Foundation
1737 H Street, NW
Washington, DC 20006
Phone (202) 223-9186

Appendix B: Select Readings

Alzheimer's Association. (1991). *Guidelines for dignity: Goals of specialized Alzheimer/dementia care in residential settings.* Chicago: Author. (available from many local chapters of the Alzheimer's Association)

Alzheimer's Association. (1995). *Activity programming for persons with dementia: A source book.* Chicago: Author.

Anderson, M.A., Beaver, K.W., & Culliton, K.C. (Eds.) (1996). *The long-term care nursing assistant training manual* (2nd ed.). Baltimore: Health Professions Press.

Aronson, M. (Ed.). (1988). *Understanding Alzheimer's disease.* New York: Charles Scribners Sons.

Bahr, M. (1992). *The memory box.* Morton Grove, IL: A. Whitman. (book for children)

Ballard, E.L. (1990). *Optimum care of the nursing home resident with Alzheimer's disease: "Give a little extra."* Durham, NC: Joseph & Kathleen Bryan Alzheimer's Disease Research Center.

Baumhover, L.A., & Beall, S.C. (Eds.). (1996). *Abuse, neglect, and exploitation of older adults: Strategies for intervention and prevention.* Baltimore: Health Professions Press.

Bell, V. (1990). Tapping an unlimited resource: Building volunteer programs for patients and their families. In N.L. Mace (Ed.), *Dementia care: Patient, family & community* (pp. 321–336). Baltimore: The Johns Hopkins University Press.

Bowlby, C. (1993). *Therapeutic activities with persons disabled by Alzheimer's disease and related disorders.* Gaithersburg, MD: Aspen Publishers.

Brawley, E.C. (1997). *Designing for Alzheimer's disease: Strategies for better care environments.* New York: John Wiley & Sons.

Chavin, M. (1991). *The lost chord: Reaching the person with dementia through the power of music.* Mt. Airy, MD: ElderSong Publications.

Clair, A.A. (1996). *Therapeutic uses of music with older adults.* Baltimore: Health Professions Press.

Coons, D., Mace, N., & Whyte, T. (1996). *Quality of life in long-term care.* New York: Haworth Press.

Couglan, P.B. (1993). *Facing Alzheimer's disease: Family caregivers speak.* New York: Ballantine Books.

Davies, P. (1988). *Grief: Climb for understanding.* New York: Lyle Stuart.

Davis, R. (1989). *My journey into Alzheimer's disease.* Wheaton, IL: Tyndale House.

Dowling, J.R. (1995). *Keeping busy: A handbook of activities for persons with dementia.* Baltimore: The Johns Hopkins University Press.

Edwards, A.J. (1994). *When memory fails: Helping the Alzheimer's and dementia patient.* New York: Plenum Press.

Feil, N. (1993). *The Validation breakthrough: Simple techniques for communicating with people with "Alzheimer's-type dementia".* Baltimore: Health Professions Press.

Guthrie, D. (1986). *Grandpa doesn't know it's me.* New York: Human Sciences Press. (book for children)

Gwyther, L. (1985). *Care of Alzheimer's patients: A manual for nursing home staff.* Chicago: American Health Care Association and Alzheimer's Association.

Hamdy, R.C. (1994). *Alzheimer's disease: A handbook for caregivers* (2nd ed.). St. Louis: C.V. Mosby.

Hellen, C.R. (1992). *Alzheimer's disease: Activity-focused care.* Andover, MA: Andover Medical Publishers.

Hoffman, S.B., & Kaplan, M. (Eds.). (1996). *Special care programs for people with dementia.* Baltimore: Health Professions Press.

Keck, D. (1996). *Forgetting whose we are: Alzheimer's disease and the love of God.* Nashville, TN: Abingdon Press.

Lindeman, D. (1991). *Alzheimer's day care: A basic guide.* New York: Hemisphere Publishing.

Mace, N.L. (1990). *Dementia care: Patient, family & community.* Baltimore: The Johns Hopkins University Press.

Mace, N.L., & Rabins, P.V. (1991). *The 36-hour day: A family guide for caring for persons with Alzheimer's disease, related dementing illnesses, and memory loss in later life* (Rev. ed.). Baltimore: The Johns Hopkins University Press.

Messenger, B. (1995). *The power of music: A complete music activities program for older adults.* Baltimore: Health Professions Press.

Morgan, B. (1992). *Alzheimer's alters us all.* Lexington, KY: Alzheimer's Association.

Office of Technology Assessment. (1987). *Losing a million minds.* Washington, DC: U.S. Government Printing Office.

Office of Technology Assessment. (1990). *Confused minds, burdened families: Finding help for people with Alzheimer's and other dementias.* Washington, DC: U.S. Government Printing Office.

Pritikin, E., & Reece, T. (1993). *Parentcare survival guide.* New York: Barron's.

Sheridan, C. (1987). *Failure free activities for the Alzheimer's patient:* A guidebook for caregivers. San Francisco: Cottage Books.

Sheridan, C. (1991). *Reminiscence: Uncovering a lifetime of memories.* San Francisco: Elder Press.

Smith, B.B., Knudson, L.A., & Bennett, M.B. (1995). *A song to set me free.* Logan, UT: Sunshine Terrace Adult Day Center.

Thews, V., Reaves, A.M., & Henry, R.S. (1993). *Now what? A handbook of activities for adult day programs.* Winston-Salem, NC: Bowman Gray School of Medicine at Wake Forest University.

Yale, R. (1995). *Developing support groups for individuals with early-stage Alzheimer's disease: Planning, implementation and evaluation.* Baltimore: Health Professions Press.

Zgola, J.M. (1987). *Doing things: A guide to programming activities for persons with Alzheimer's disease and related disorders.* Baltimore: The Johns Hopkins University Press.

Appendix C: Our Best Friends

The authors share some favorite memories of their "Best Friends" featured throughout the book. We thank the individuals involved and their families for giving us permission to tell their stories.

Jean Leslie Auxier (1899–1994)

Jean learned to read before starting school. His method of learning was to say to any adult, "I bet you don't know what this word is," and he would add another word to his vocabulary. He learned to read so well that he began school in the third grade.

Known as the "best judge Pike County ever produced," he was appointed U.S. Attorney for the Eastern District of Kentucky by President Dwight D. Eisenhower. Jean was not only a good judge but also a humanitarian, known for helping others. He sometimes gave the coat he was wearing to a needy client.

He enjoyed traveling, big game hunting, and American history. At the day center, the Judge enjoyed reading aloud about American presidents, but only about the Republicans!

Joe Blackhurst (1906–   )

"Glasgow belongs to me," Joe sings of his place of birth, Glasgow, Scotland. Joe's gift of music is in his genes. He has a song for every occasion, from the hymns of his church to funny ditties he often sang in community musicals and entertaining old friends. He would rather dance than eat!

Joe's wife, Bessie, now deceased; his two sons, Edward and Eric; and their families have always been his greatest joy. Joe takes special pride in the fact that he always worked hard and at the same time provided volunteer service to the community, earning the Silver Beaver Award for his Boy Scout endeavors. He enjoyed being a lay reader in his church and managed to make time for sports and gardening. Joe has a wonderful sense of humor and a contagious love of life.

Margaret Hayes Brubaker (1907–1996)

Margaret was born in Duluth, Minnesota, and moved to California at an early age. There she graduated from the famous Hollywood High. In an era when many women worked only in the home, Margaret

---

The biographies were completed in August 1996.

worked in a variety of positions, including a family-owned restaurant and her father's ice cream company.

Margaret and her late husband, Dudley, raised their son, James ("Jim"), in a neighborhood full of his cousins. The Brubakers lived next door to Dudley's sister and brother-in-law, Lois and Siegfried ("Sig") Haas, with whom they had a 60-year friendship. Margaret was proud of Jim and his career as a movie producer and of her grand-children Marcei, Susan, and John.

Even late in her illness, Margaret remained interested and in-volved in the world around her. Her family remembers her as a "take-charge" person with a wonderful sense of humor.

Mary Burmaster (1914–)

"My name is pronounced "*Bur*-master" not "Bur-*master*," Mary, a quiet, thoughtful person, makes clear.

Famous American and English writers are no strangers to Mary because she is often the first to finish a familiar line from one of their works. When her daughter Betsey was a little girl, Mary taught her the poem that she learned when she was a little girl. She enjoys sharing with us the Betsey version: "The Northwind doth blow and we shall have snow. What will poor robin do then? He'll sit in the barn to keep himself warm and tuck his head under his wing. Poor 'shing' [instead of 'thing']."

Mary knows every word to the songs of the big band era. Nothing pleases her more than to sing throughout the day, unless it is to talk about her three children Lee, Betsey, and Mary Anne.

Ruby Lee Chiles (1918–)

"Let's get busy with all this work to do. I like to get my work done early and then sit back." These words demonstrate Ruby Lee's strong work ethic, one of the key elements of her life story. She might also say, "Just bring it here, I'll fix it. I'm used to working hard."

Ruby is very proud of her family; she likes to talk about lessons learned from her parents and how she passed these on to her four children.

Ruby is friendly and compassionate. She likes to help others and is ready to console those who need support. She can write beautiful words of encouragement on cards to send to others. She would love nothing better than to take all of her Best Friends home with her for a big party.

Christine Clark (1916–1992)

"I'll make you some chicken and dumplin's, Honey. You'll love my dumplin's." Christine spent a lifetime cooking for others, including her family of nine siblings, then in her own home, her church, and at her job. At age 14, Christine began working as a live-in cook and housekeeper.

Christine was devoted to her family—her husband, two daughters, Linda and Wanneta; grandchildren; and great-grandchildren—and her church, the First Baptist Church in Nicholasville, Kentucky. She was easygoing, appreciative, cooperative, and kind.

The students at the day center who knew her always appreciated her loving, encouraging hugs.

Vernon "Vern" Clark (1927–1996)

Vern Clark was born in Glendale, California, and was close to his parents and sister. He owned a trucking business, and his wife, Carolyn, and three children Kathy, Pam, and Lori remember him as a hard worker with high standards.

After retiring from his trucking business, he and Carolyn bought the Ocean Palms Motel in Pismo Beach, California. Vern took tremendous pride in the motel, and his family recall Vern's disappointment whenever guests did not take proper care of their room.

When Vern became ill with Alzheimer's disease, the adult day center he attended was a source of many new friends and much joy. He also enjoyed visits from his six grandchildren and one great-grandchild. Although Vern could be quiet and rather shy around strangers, he always "lit up" around his family, often displaying his great sense of humor.

Tennessee "Tennie" S. Clayton (1904–1989)

A good student and winner of her school's spelling bee, Tennie embraced a lifelong love of learning. After marriage, she worked hard on the family farm cooking, canning, sewing, quilting, and caring for three children, Gretchen, Catherine, and Buddy.

She always designed and made clothes for herself, the children, and other family members and friends. Because money was scarce, she made her own patterns and often used material from feed sacks for sewing. Her family, her friends, and her church spelled happiness for Tennie.

She enjoyed reminiscing about her early childhood, especially about growing up with a cousin, Roxie, who was just like a twin sister.

Her friends described her as pleasant, reserved, and a bit shy. With her snow-white hair pulled back in a tight bun and her old-fashioned print dresses, she often looked like a figure in a Norman Rockwell painting.

Brevard Crihfield (1916–1987)

Brevard, nicknamed "Crihf," took enormous pride in being reminded of his past as Executive Director of the Council of State Governments. Friends and family could remember him staying busy in various committee meetings or enjoying a break with a newspaper, a cup of coffee, and a cigarette.

Crihf's early years were spent in Illinois, and he recalled "Ronnie" Reagan attending Eureka College in Illinois while he attended the University of Chicago. Family, his dog "Ho," beautiful art books, and favorite poems were also topics of conversation. Another interest was baseball; he played second base like a pro.

Crihf was a very private person. When he enrolled in the Helping Hand Day Center, he approached most activities cautiously, yet he was a superb dancer and would always embrace an opportunity to dance, especially to the music of Benny Goodman's orchestra.

Mary Katherine Davis (1907–1992)

When Mary Katherine enrolled in the Helping Hand Day Center in Lexington, Kentucky, she insisted on being called "Mickey," the nickname given to her when she attended nurses' training in Charleston, West Virginia. After graduation, Mickey specialized in caring for trauma patients and loved her profession. She was a nurse through and through.

During her youth, she disliked many aspects of living on a farm, although she did enjoy the wide open spaces, the trees and flowers, and the stream running through the farm. She enjoyed reading and keeping up with news of the outside world, an interest that stayed with her.

Mickey was small in stature but big in spirit, which she shared with her family and friends, her career, and her church.

Rubena S. Dean (1931–   )

"The Yellow Rose of Texas" brings a big smile to Rubena's face as she recalls many happy memories of her childhood in Texas and her graduation from Texas University for Women in Denton. She loved her years of teaching physical education, English, and history to junior high school students.

Rubena enjoys being part of a large extended family and maintains close relationships with her children, Lynn and Ted, and her grandchildren. Helping people has also been a major part of her life. Her community benefited from her giving spirit; she was president of many service-related clubs, she organized church activities, and she volunteered in nursing facilities. Rubena thrived on hard work. Before onset of her illness, she enjoyed hobbies such as playing bridge and piano and needlepoint.

Edna Denton Edwards (1909–   )

Edna is proud to be part of a tradition of three generations of third-grade teachers; she followed her mother, and her daughter Peggy followed her. Edna has many talents; she is an artist (her artwork is on the cover of *Activity Programming for Persons with Dementia: A Source Book*, noted in Appendix B), a pianist, a seamstress, and a good cook, known for making an excellent corn pudding.

After her husband died, Edna was both mother and father to their three daughters Patricia, Peggy, and Janet. The Immanuel Baptist Church remains her tower of strength.

Edna is highly competitive, is a big tease, loves to clown around, and makes friends easily.

Marydean Evans (1910–   )

"Did you really 'pogo' down Broadway and in the front window of your father's sporting goods store?" a friend of Marydean's once asked in disbelief. Marydean's father had the latest equipment, including the first pogo stick in Kentucky. She and her four brothers and sisters helped publicize this new contraption.

Swimming, dancing (she was known as the best dancer at the famous Brown Hotel's Roof Garden in Louisville, Kentucky), and preparing fancy food as a caterer are some of Marydean's accomplishments. Chocolate in any form is a favorite food, and butter is a close second. "Bread is just a vehicle to deliver butter," she admits with a grin.

Marydean is a cheerful person. Her children, Betty, Tip, and Ann, and her grandchildren provide strong support. They are proud of her volunteer work to help others.

Henrietta Frazier (1921–   )

"Our house has always been for everyone." Henrietta is proud that her house was home base for family and friends. The youngest of six children, she enjoyed all the comings and goings in a close extended family. With a nursing degree from St. Elizabeth's Hospital School of Nursing, Henrietta served both the private and public sectors in a caring, thoughtful, and dedicated manner.

When she was 4 years old, Henrietta had to have an eye removed. Despite her vision impairment, she has embraced life fully. She has a jolly disposition, with a quick wit.

She and her sister, Mae, have traveled extensively and especially enjoy cruises. Because they live together, they share many close friends. Henrietta is an avid fan of basketball, and a joiner of clubs and causes.

Sergio ("Serge") Torres Gajardo (1920–1995)

Serge was always a big tease! "I left Chile because one day when I was piloting a small plane, I swooped down over a chicken coop, crashed my plane, and killed all the chickens." Serge was a second lieutenant in the Chilean Air Force before becoming an American citizen.

His family included his wife, Gertrude; their three children, Roxanne, Suzi, and John; and three grandchildren. They vacationed together in a favorite spot in Mexico and were active in all aspects of their church.

Music was woven into Serge's life in many ways. He loved to dance to the rhythms of Latin music. He enjoyed a wide range of songs, from big band tunes to classical and opera. Playing tennis and ping-pong and following the Chicago Cubs and the Green Bay Packers gave him great pleasure. He also liked to fish, hunt, swim, and read. Serge was affectionate, unselfish, and full of fun.

Edna Carroll Greenwade (1916–1996)

Edna Carroll grew up on a farm, the youngest of five brothers and sisters. Edna Carroll enjoyed being teased: "Did your brothers and sisters spoil you?" She denied being spoiled, but in fact had many memories of being the "baby doll" in the family. Her daughter Katie, grandchildren, and one great-grandson were central to her life.

Helpfulness and caring about others was a great part of Edna Carroll's life. She was active in her church, helping to cook special dinners. A library of recipes stood ready for her to share a dish of food for any occasion. She enjoyed sewing, quilting, and working with ceramics. A loving person, Edna Carroll was anxious to please, friendly, and fun.

Geri Greenway (1940–   )

"That is van Gogh's *The Starry Night*," Geri might quickly point out when leafing through a beautiful book of paintings. The worlds of art, literature, and opera are familiar territory for her. Impressively, she reads about those subjects in several languages.

Earning a Ph.D. in German literature, she taught at several colleges. She endeared herself to her students with her extensive knowledge and her ability to teach her subjects in a relaxed atmosphere of learning.

Geri is proud of her family; together they enjoyed traveling, swimming, gardening, and jogging. Adopting a whale named Olympia was just one expression of Geri's ecological concern. She enjoys Cajun food, a taste treat from her birth state of Louisiana. Talented, sophisticated, beautiful, and loving describe Geri.

Pauline G. Huffman (1914–   )

Pauline was called a "tomboy" when she was growing up. Instead of playing with dolls befitting little girls at that time, she preferred to play ball with her brothers. She has always liked sports of all kinds, especially tennis, baseball, basketball, football, and bowling. When not playing sports, Pauline enjoyed attending games or watching them on television.

Pauline made many clothes for herself and friends, played the piano, and was an avid worker of crossword puzzles. Her family is central to her life; her husband, her son and his wife, a granddaughter, and one great-grandson are her first love. Pauline stands up for what she thinks is right, but always with a winning smile.

Dicy Bell Reed Jenkins (1902–1991)

Born in the Oklahoma Territory before Oklahoma became a state, Dicy liked to recall her early childhood living in tents and in covered wagons. She bragged that she could do everything her eight brothers did, including chopping and hauling wood and working in the fields.

Dicy amazed everyone with her catalog of old sayings. When asked how she was feeling, she always said, "A little better than a blank." Other expressions that she used often were "No fool, no fun," "mother wit," and "there's no fool like an old fool." Feisty at times, shaking her cane to make a point, Dicy still endeared herself to everyone.

Dicy and her husband, Lawrence, had two children, Lawrencetta and Edward, and raised two granddaughters, Nawanta and Nelvean. Dicy lived with Nawanta during the last years of her life. A devoted family and a strong faith in God sustained Dicy through good and bad times.

Betty Justice (1927–   )

Betty's face is a "picture show" of communication, lighting up with a contagious smile when she greets friends or family members. She has always been a happy person, juggling her many responsibilities with ease. She cared for the animals on the farm, worked as a nursing assistant in a local facility, and is "Mom" to four children. Her family, including children, grandchildren, and great-grandchildren, is the pride of her life, but her husband, Bill, gets the biggest hug. The death of their only son is a source of sadness only parents can understand.

Betty is very musical, singing old gospel songs taught to her by her minister grandfather, humming while she works, and dancing at the drop of a hat.

Leota Kilkenny (1903–1994)

"St. John, Kentucky. That's close to Louisville." Leota enjoyed recalling her early years on the farm near St. John. The boys milked the cows, and the milk was shipped by train to Louisville. She had vivid memories of being invited to ride to the station and watch as the milk was loaded on the train. She loved the farm, especially the animals and the woods near the house, where she played with many brothers and sisters. Leota graduated from high school at nearby Bethlehem Academy.

A full-time homemaker, Leota was a dedicated wife and mother of three children, Ann Marie, John, and Mary Jane. She and her family were active in the Roman Catholic church. Always ready to give a hug, she was kind, thoughtful, and fun-loving.

Helen C. King (1921–   )

"I want to feel that I am learning new information or doing something useful. I hate busy work." Helen's background of being a teacher and librarian shines through. She wants a challenge.

Helen lights up the room when she arrives. She is interested and interesting. Demonstrating dances such as the *Charleston,* storytelling, drawing, and painting in an abstract form are her special talents. At her day center, she is chief enthusiast for the "word of the day" based on the letters of the alphabet. She chooses words such as "oxymoron."

Compassionate and concerned about others, Helen is pure joy.

Masanori "Mas" Matsumura (1937–   )

Born in Santa Monica, California, "Mas" Matsumura was the oldest of three children and part of a close-knit family. He was 5 years old when his family was interned in Manzanar, California, during World War II. Notably, the photographer Ansel Adams took his portrait during that time. As a young man, Mas was very athletic and motivated.

He has been married to his wife, May, for over 35 years. They have three children, Cindy, Donna, and Riki. Before retiring in 1993, he worked in a commercial nursery business that specializes in gardenias.

His children say that Mas is always there for them. "A friendly and gentle spirit" is a description that comes to mind whenever one thinks of Mas.

Willa Lee McCabe (1915–   )

"Sometime the little ones cried on the first day of school. I just hugged and hugged them." Willa, a first-grade teacher for 32 years, knew exactly what to do. Children, including her grandsons Greg and Jason, are the light of Willa's life.

Willa enjoys talking about the past, including the fun she had walking to school with her friends, taking her school lunch in a straw lunch basket, and playing games at recess. She also enjoys talking about her special hobbies, including raising a vegetable garden and making quilts, listening to music, singing, and taking long walks. Willa's face shows a contagious burst of joy when greeting friends. She lights up the room, energizing the people around her.

Thelma Lydia Berner Moody (1911–   )

When friends and family think of Thelma, what comes to mind first is her lifelong love of children and nature. She loved to encourage children to listen to the thunder and feel the wind of a storm to better understand the natural world. Thelma always taught her family and others about the stars in the sky; life in the sea, lakes, streams, and ponds; and the geology of the Earth. As a teacher at the Buffalo (New

York) Museum of Natural Science, Thelma introduced many children to the wonders of the natural sciences.

She was enthusiastically committed to her family, giving love and attention to husband, Julian, and children Linda, Julian, and Laurie. Everyone knows Thelma as a woman of great honesty, compassion, and enthusiasm for life.

Ruby Mae Morris (1912–   )

A life of hard work did not dampen Ruby Mae's love of having a good time. She is a prankster and always loves a good joke.

Her love of children and animals is evident: "God gave them to us to love and care for," she reminds us often. Her family, her church, and caring for others are central to her life. Ruby Mae insists that she does not mind hard work: "Just get the paint and I'll paint your house all the way to the roof. I can do lots of things that you don't know about." She loves to sing and dance and stays dressed in her best clothes, "camera-ready," for her picture to be taken.

Her daughter, Dolores, praises her: "She's a very special rose in our garden and God will pick her for an eternal garden." She has a sweet, sweet spirit.

Larkin Myers (1910–1993)

Larkin Myers, affectionately known to his friends and family as "Myers," loved nothing better than to "chew the fat" over a cup of coffee with his friends. Tales from his days as a policeman entertained everyone. He was often kidded by friends, saying, "I must watch my step or Myers will put me in jail!" Kind, thoughtful, affectionate, and fun-loving, he did not fit many people's image of a rather stern policeman. Friends also enjoyed talking about his responsibilities as the man in charge of all the traffic signal coordination in Lexington.

Myers and his wife, Chris, had the joy of their niece, Dana, and her mother coming to live with them when Dana was 3 years old. Myers loved children, and he and Dana, whom he called "Sug," were buddies. Dana praises him: "I was so influenced by his genuine caring attitude."

Patsy Peck (1927–   )

Patsy is a nature enthusiast; she can identify many birds by their songs and is knowledgeable about animals and their homes and habits. She was pleased when a friend said to her, "I saw your favorite bird, the puffin, while visiting in the Orkney Islands." She has worked to protect the environment for future generations.

Her love of nature is surpassed only by her love of children. She is never too busy to spend time with a child; it may be just a hug or hours of reassuring play.

A graduate of Stevens College in Missouri, Patsy organized the physical therapy program for a local hospital. She was a dedicated, fun-loving administrator, always ready to help others.

Marcus P. Powell (1911–1994)

A professor in Environmental Health and Preventive Medicine at the University of Iowa, Marcus Powell led a life of dedication to his family and students. He mentored many students who earned master's and doctorate degrees under his direction, and took a particular interest in students from other countries. Although he had high expectations of his students, more than one student took an exam over because Marcus felt he or she deserved another try.

Called "Papa" by his family, he was devoted to his wife, Ethel, and children Mark and Carmen. Some of the hobbies Marcus enjoyed included fishing, small-game hunting, and growing African violets and show-quality roses. He even had a totem pole collection!

"Papa" is best remembered for his compassion for others and passion for learning. He embraced life to the fullest.

Jerome ("Jerry") Ruttenberg (1908–1987)

A series of small strokes could not steal all of Jerry's sense of humor and amazing intellect. He had a pun for almost every occasion, and his quick wit brought joy to all. Once when he heard the song "Cruising Down the River" being sung off-key, Jerry was quick to say, "Lifeboats, please, we're sinking." In answer to the question "What do you remember about being 12 years old?" he quipped, "Waiting to be 13."

He named his favorite dog "Sooner," telling all that he chose this name because the dog would "rather eat sooner than later." Dancing, singing, card games, and word puzzles spelled relaxation for him. Jerry was an outstanding businessman, a humanitarian, an avid reader, and most of all, a devoted husband and father.

Howard Fenimore Shipps (1903–1992)

The word "commitment" sums up the life of Dr. Howard Shipps. He was committed to his religious faith, his family, and his profession. A

minister and a professor, a gardener and a sports enthusiast, a grandfather and a great-grandfather, he had a wide range of interests and
abilities.

He pursued additional professional studies before it became popular, and in retirement continued his interest in books, music, travel,
his collection of beautiful glassware and old tools, and antique furniture refinishing. Howard was deliberate and thoughtful of speech.
He did not speak often, but when he spoke he had something to say,
often exposing his dry wit. He was a gentleman and a gentle man to
the very end of his life.

Evelyn Merrell Talbott (1913–1992)

Evelyn was known as a bookworm even as a little girl; as she grew up
her books were her best friends. At the day center she would often
announce, "I brought a new book for us to enjoy today." Soon she
would be immersed in a book, such as *The Wonders of the Underwater
World*. She turned this love of books into a degree in library science
from the University of Kentucky. She enjoyed working as a librarian
for many years.

Evelyn's dog, Willie, was very much a part of her family, which
included her husband, Bob, and their daughter, Susan. Willie even
traveled with the family; a favorite trip was going to the beach. Evelyn
loved music and dancing. She was always friendly and appreciative.

Walter Turner (1913–1993)

"Come here! Let me see your pretty picture." Walter adored children
and they always gave Walter their affectionate smiles. Walter and his
wife, Mable, had 14 children, so Walter was an "old pro" with little
ones.

Walter often bragged that his family was almost self-sufficient
living on top of Pine Mountain in eastern Kentucky. They grew all
their vegetables; cultivated a fruit and berry orchard; raised chickens,
turkeys, hogs, and cattle for meat; tended bees for honey; and grew
cane for sorghum. He could describe in detail how to make "moon-
shine." Walter worked hard as a coal miner. He was especially proud
of being able to educate his children while passing on to them many
mountain traditions.

Beverly Wheeler (1936–   )

Beverly was born in Ventura, California. Beverly's friends and family
describe her as a good and loyal friend who has always been very
organized, precise, and goal-oriented. She and her husband, Michael,

have been married for over 38 years and have two sons, Kelly and Chris.

Beverly is proud of her 17-year teaching career, working with children from kindergarten to sixth grade. She has long had an interest in quilting, and is considered to be very artistic, with an excellent sense of color and design.

Since her diagnosis of Alzheimer's disease, Beverly made a film (*My Challenge with Alzheimer's Disease*) describing her experiences and has spoken at classes and seminars. Her family remain proud of her courage in facing Alzheimer's disease.

Marian Wilks Witte (1903–1993)

Marian drove the first car in her hometown of Verona, Missouri, and liked to say that there was always a handsome man close by to "crank" the car. One of her first jobs was copying laws by longhand in huge law books at the Missouri state capitol.

Marian swam often as a child and continued to swim all her life. She loved to sing, whistle, read stories about animals, and talk about her family.

Words and phrases such as "jovial," "lovable," and "devoted to family and friends" describe Marian. "I'm Marian Witte, but I'm not very witty," she would often say, exposing her sense of humor, which must have been a bright spot for the patients she sat with until she was almost 80 years old.

Emma Parido Woods (1921–1992)

Emma grew up with three brothers who took good care of her when she was a little girl. After high school, she worked in the tobacco industry in the "re-drier" where tobacco was processed for shipping, and as a time keeper. That was hard work, Emma could attest to that!

On June 4, 1950, Emma married Howard Woods. Together they raised eight children. The parental terms of endearment given to them by the children were "Big Momma" and "Big Daddy." Emma became a full-time homemaker, and their house became the gathering place for all, including grandchildren and great-grandchildren. Emma was devoted to her family. She also maintained a strong religious faith, enjoying listening to and singing hymns.

Nancy Zechman (1928–1992)

A very athletic person during her youth, Nancy chose to major in physical education at Miami University in Oxford, Ohio. Her athletic interest and ability continued throughout her life, and she had a special skill and flair for tennis.

Nancy was also an artistic person, creating a beautiful home for her husband, Fred, children Rick and Jami; and her cats Marilyn and Monroe. She volunteered on a regular basis at a local hospital and pursued many other interests including attending art classes and workshops, gardening, playing cards, doing needlework, and playing sports of all varieties.

Nancy's infectious smile and love of people kept her surrounded with "friends aplenty."

Index

Page numbers followed by "f" indicate figures; page numbers followed by "t" indicate tables.

Alzheimer's disease, *see*
Identity confusion; Time
confusion
Control, sense of, importance of in
persons with Alzheimer's
disease, 133
Crihfield, Brevard, 15, 82, 228
CT, *see* Computed tomography
Cues, misreading, 97, 98
Currie, Rodger, 51

Davis, Mary Katherine, 81, 228
Dean, Rubena, 13, 58, 228
Delusions, 16
Dementia
AIDS and, 5
causes of, 22
defined, 6
multi-infarct, 5
Parkinson's disease and, 5
treatable causes of, 23
visuospatial perception and, 15
Denial, 168
Depression, 13, 22
Dewhirst, Gary, 57
Diagnosis, importance of
knowledge of in *persons*
with Alzheimer's disease,
39, 144
Disabilities, excess
defined, 25
reducing, 29
Distraction, use of with *persons*
with Alzheimer's disease,
108, 110, 111, 121–122
Drugs
challenging behavior,
moderating, 24, 40
experimental studies, and
memory disorder clinics,
158
use of in Alzheimer's disease,
115

Durable power of attorney, 23

Educational background of *person*
with Alzheimer's disease,
knowledge of, 67, 70, 73
Edwards, Edna, 52, 55–56, 229
EEG, *see* Electroencephalogram
Elder abuse intervention services,
157
Electroencephalogram (EEG), 23
Embarrassment, feelings of in
persons with Alzheimer's
disease, 12t, 17, 57
Environment, living
communication, facilitating in,
117
safe, structured, and predictable,
importance of in *persons*
with Alzheimer's disease,
40
simplifying, 112, 146
Evans, Marydean, 48, 57, 229
Expectations, realistic, 27–28, 96,
99–100, 145

Families, 4
and adult day services,
reluctance to use, 168–169
encouraging use of, 169,
171–172
and Alzheimer's Disease Bill of
Rights, 150
assessment form, using, 30–31
as caregivers, 150
in crisis, 2
decision making of, dynamics in,
172
support groups for, 2, 24
Fear, feelings of in *persons* with
Alzheimer's disease, 12t,
15–16

Nicknames of *person* with Alzheimer's disease, knowledge of, 69
Nursing assistants, *see* Home health aides
Nursing facilities
family members' emotional problems with, 179–180
placement in, 157, 191–192
role of in expanding caregiving network, 84
staff, 4
recasting relationships with *persons* with Alzheimer's disease, 62–63
"three hugs a day" rule, 61
Nutritional programs, 157

Paranoia, feelings of in *persons* with Alzheimer's disease, 12*t*, 16
Parents and grandparents of *person* with Alzheimer's disease, knowledge of, 67
Parkinson's disease, and dementia, 5, 22
Peck, Patsy, 82–83, 235
Personal care, as activity, 134
Personal growth, importance of in *persons* with Alzheimer's disease, 133
Personality, pre- and postmorbid, understanding, 29, 33–34, 74–75
Personality changes, and Alzheimer's disease, 21, 22
Pets, of *person* with Alzheimer's disease
being with as activity, 135
knowledge of, 70
Physical contact, importance of in *persons* with Alzheimer's disease, 41
Physical health, assessment of, 28

Pick's disease, and dementia, 22
Planning, "knack" of coping with upsets in, 107
Play, importance of in *persons* with Alzheimer's disease, 131
Points of Life Foundation, The, 220
Powell, Marcus P., 54, 235
Preferences of *person* with Alzheimer's disease, knowledge of, 74
Present, focusing on, 146
Problem-solving ability, and Alzheimer's disease, 21, 22
Productivity, importance of in *persons* with Alzheimer's disease, 39, 131
Psychotropic medications, 25
freedom from, importance of in *persons* with Alzheimer's disease, 40

Questions
open-ended, importance of use of with *persons* with Alzheimer's disease, 106
overwhelming, "knack" of coping with, 105–106
Quiet time, enjoying, as activity, 138–139, 146

Reagan, Ronald, 2, 228
Relationships, recasting
for family caregivers, 61–62, 101, 145–146
for professional caregivers, 62–63, 101
Reminiscing, as activity, 136, 152
Repetition, "knack" of coping with, 110–111
Respite care, 23, 125–126, 158
Retirement of *person* with

About the Authors

Virginia Bell, M.S.W., has developed an international reputation for her unique sensitivity to *persons* with Alzheimer's disease. She has challenged many people to rethink their approaches to dementia care, in part through her development of the Helping Hand Adult Day Center (sponsored by the Lexington/Bluegrass chapter of the Alzheimer's Association) in Lexington, Kentucky, one of the first dementia-specific adult day programs and one of the best. In 1994 she was awarded the prestigious Ruth Von Behren Award from the National Council on Aging for her work in programming and excellence in day care settings.

She has published in the field of Alzheimer's disease and lectured throughout the world, including eight presentations at Alzheimer's Disease International conferences. Ms. Bell was funded (along with David Troxel) by the Robert Wood Johnson Foundation to take part in the foundation's Dementia Care and Respite Services program, the first major initiative and study to evaluate and encourage the expansion of adult day services in the United States.

After retiring from the University of Kentucky Sanders-Brown Center on Aging, Ms. Bell volunteered full-time in the Helping Hand program, where she coordinates the volunteer programs. She can be reached at the Alzheimer's Association, Lexington/Bluegrass Chapter, 801 South Limestone, Suite E, Lexington, Kentucky 40508, or by e-mail at VBellKY@aol.com.

David Troxel, M.P.H., began his work in Alzheimer's disease in 1986 at the University of Kentucky Sanders-Brown Center on Aging, then one of only 10 federally funded Alzheimer's disease research centers. He, Virginia Bell, and others established a statewide network of support groups and services for Kentuckians with Alzheimer's disease and their caregivers.

He was the first executive director of the Lexington/Bluegrass chapter of the Alzheimer's Association, and with Virginia Bell, won an unprecedented four Excellence in Program Awards for patient and family services, the annual award given to local Alzheimer's Association chapters by the national association.

Mr. Troxel has written and lectured widely about Alzheimer's disease. He cowrote (with Virginia Bell) "An Alzheimer's Disease Bill of Rights," which first appeared in 1995 and has been extensively reprinted and has been translated into a dozen languages.

He has been active in the leadership of the American Public Health Association and is the Executive Director of the Santa Barbara chapter of the Alzheimer's Association. He can be reached at that office at 2024 De La Vina Street, Santa Barbara, California 93105, or by e-mail at SBDAVIDT@aol.com.

Health Professions Press Titles of Related Interest

❖ **Best Friends** (20-minute VHS videocassette), produced by the Stone Advisory for the Lexington/Bluegrass (KY) Alzheimer's Association
❖ **Caring for People with Alzheimer's Disease: A Training Manual for Direct Care Providers**, by Gayle Andresen, R.N.-C., M.S., A.N.P./G.N.P., in association with Health Education Development System, Inc., and Cooperative Health Education Program (HEDS/CHEP)
❖ **Developing Support Groups for Individuals with Early-Stage Alzheimer's Disease: Planning, Implementation, and Evaluation**, by Robyn Yale, L.C.S.W.
❖ **The Validation Breakthrough: Simple Techniques for Communicating with People with "Alzheimer's-Type Dementia,"** by Naomi Feil, M.S.W.
❖ **Special Care Programs for People with Dementia**, edited by Stephanie B. Hoffman, Ph.D., and Mary Kaplan, M.S.W.
❖ **Breaking Through Dementia** (90-minute audiocassette), produced by Scott Averill
❖ **Abuse, Neglect, and Exploitation of Older Persons: Strategies for Assessment and Intervention**, edited by Lorin Baumhover, Ph.D., and S. Colleen Beall, Dr.P.H.
❖ **Older Adulthood: Learning Activities for Understanding Aging**, by Stephen Fried, Ph.D., et al.
❖ **More than Movement for Fit to Frail Older Adults: Creative Activities for the Body, Mind, and Spirit**, by Pauline Fisher, M.A.
❖ **The Power of Music: A Complete Music Activities Program for Older Adults**, by Bill Messenger, M.L.A.
❖ **Therapeutic Caregiving: A Practical Guide for Caregivers of Persons with Alzheimer's and Other Dementia Causing Diseases**, by Barbara Bridges, R.N., M.S.N., M.S.H.C.M., M.B.A.

For further information on these and other titles, or to receive a free catalog, call, write, or e-mail the HPP customer service department.

The Best Friends Approach to Alzheimer's Care

*Do you know someone with whom you would like to share
the Best Friends method?*

To order additional copies of **The Best Friends Approach to
Alzheimer's Care**, simply complete the information below and
send to Health Professions Press.

Ordering Information

YES! Please send me _____ copies of **The Best Friends Approach to
Alzheimer's Care** at $24.95 each. (price subject to change)

❏ Check or money order enclosed (payable to Health Professions Press)

❏ Bill my institution (attach purchase order)

❏ MasterCard ❏ VISA ❏ American Express

Exp. date _____ / _____ Card no. _____

Signature _____

Name _____

Address _____

City/State/Zip _____

Daytime telephone (___) _____ ZBF

❏ Please send me a copy of your current catalog

**HEALTH
PROFESSIONS
PRESS**

Health Professions Press   (888) 337-8808 (toll free)
P.O. Box 10624
Baltimore, MD 21285-0624

For *fast* delivery, *fax* your order to: (410) 337-8539
Or e-mail to: hpp@pbrookes.com